TRAFFICKING

How Chronic Inflammation Sabotages the Immune Arsenal
and Poisons the Interstitial Space of End Organs

ROBERT L BUCKINGHAM, MD, FACP

ISBN: 978-1-963068-37-5 (hc)
ISBN: 978-1-963068-35-1 (sc)
ISBN: 978-1-963068-36-8 (e)

Library of Congress Control Number: 2024904863

R Buckingham MD, FACP

TABLE OF CONTENTS

INTRODUCTION

Chronic inflammation is the dark energy in all interstitial spaces. Our poor lifestyle choices fuel it but we don't expect its arrival. And when symptoms appear the fatigue and pain they cause are relentless. We can't help but break down from the weight of the chronic inflammatory avalanche on our bodies and psyche. No end organ is spared as weight accumulates, and blood pressure, sugar and LDL cholesterol levels increase. In our busy and chaotic lives, we *don't* make the connection of these mid -life add-ons to chronic fatigue, achy knees, blurred vision, hearing loss, root canals, brain fog, or sleep deprivation. From combinations of denial, shock and stupor we are thrust into the medical industrial complex and the sudden volleys of replacement surgeries, stents, bypass grafts and the removal of sick and bloated gallbladders. Prescription medications proliferate to treat depression, anxiety, insomnia, pain, rheumatic diseases, hypertension, diabetes, and lipid disorders. We don't like the way we feel or look but we accept our plight of chronic pain and fatigue. Meanwhile chronic inflammation is having a heyday in our interstitial spaces. By age 60, many of us have given up, content to find solace on the couch, curled up with a dog, bag of chips and a television or cell phone to keep us company.

What becomes uncanny is how bad behavior feeds on itself. The couch and chips could lead to a long nap, a beer two or three or a bag of cookies. All of these choices are reactive, as they feed a chain reaction of addictions triggered by sugar and salt. The long daytime nap feeds nighttime insomnia, which will also trigger use of sleeping pills and midnight sugar snacking. Without a clue we have invited chronic inflammation into our interstitial spaces and it is bringing us to our knees with one poor choice after another. Before we can say helter-skelter, we are ensconced in disease treatment, surgeries and imaging studies. Everything gets harder, from thinking to getting out of a chair. Life suddenly seems unfair as odds and choices are stacked against us. And short of pills, more tests and surgeries, nobody seems to have a clue as to how to get out of this hole. We feel doomed and want comfort.

What we have to acknowledge is that most of what is offered by the medical establishment is stop-gap. We have to resist the tendency for a quick fix and realize the fix must come from our own choices. While drugs, imaging and surgery can be lifesaving and have their place, in the grand scheme of things, they t mirror disease *treatment* and don't solve the problem of disease *prevention*. In other words, we never get to the point of stopping the chronic inflammatory train and getting off.

Yet that is exactly what we must do to get healthy. To become less reactionary and more intentional about how we live. This means no double talk about addictions, exercise, sleep, diet or how much stress we place ourselves sunder. Consciously choices should be made on the basis of do they increase or decrease inflammation? In most cases this becomes self- explanatory. When we base choice on outcomes, we have transitioned from being reactionary to becoming intentional. Good things will happen. Suddenly wellness and prevention instead of disease treatment become passwords to our subliminal conscious.

Making matters worse, is that our health care providers may actually be antagonizing our efforts to change. As providers, we don't get paid to spend time with patients to teach the right and wrong of lifestyle. Instead we get paid and rewarded for prescribing drugs for disease treatment and for timely referrals, procedures and injections to hunt for and treat more disease. Wellness and disease prevention are still mostly foreign concepts to the volume driven and employed primary care physician. As we open our prescription pads to treat disease we ignore the chronic inflammatory elephant in the room, which is stemming the disease we are treating.

The implication is that treating diseases is a *late outcome* of chronic inflammation (see graph 3 appendix). At the disease treatment stage, chronic inflammation has already capsized the interstitial space to its own liking. The capillary cells, which compose the smallest of blood vessels, have decomposed to the point where they no longer have capacity to control the trafficking whereabouts of immune arsenal entering or leaving interstitial spaces. This breakdown has produced an opportunity for chronic inflammation to birth. Over time and fueled with vascular inflammatory free radicals seeding into interstitial spaces, chronic inflammation harnesses its own set of alternative feedback loops provided by immune arsenal gone wrong. These loops displace those of the weakened capillary cell to create its own agenda, which is proinflammatory and anti-end organ. It is this maturing of chronic inflammation within the interstitial space that enables the proliferation of end organ disease venues that we as health care providers have learned so well to treat. Unbeknownst to both provider and patient is that without acknowledging prevention, we are losing the disease treatment battle. Meanwhile ever increasingly expensive technologies, drugs and surgeries weave their way into disease treatment in an ever increasing spiral of expensive treatments. The trouble is that diseases adapt and always seem to be at least one step ahead of our prescription pads. The proliferation will be endless and will lead to bankrupting the medical establishment. I can't tell which is worse, the greed from incentive induced providers, or from nervous patients, who want all the latest imaging and surgery in the hopes of finding the silver bullet.

This is where wellness steps in. In this model, lifestyle adjustments block chronic interstitial space inflammation by reducing vascular inflammatory free radicals. Disease venues are prevented before they start. Or in some cases, with their fuel source exhausted, they dry up. Interstitial space feedback loop momentum shifts back to the capillary cell as they come out of hibernation and resume their pivot and swing dance. That is capillary cell outer membranes begin to once again *choreograph* immune arsenal trafficking into interstitial spaces, which increases the likelihood of successful interstitial space inflammatory breach removal, which then enables the swinging of mitochondrial combustion from energy to nitric oxide. Interstitial space wellness has made a comeback!

Pushing back against chronic inflammatory momentum is much easier to accomplish if attempted earlier in the game. By limiting the vascular inflammatory free radical fuel source much earlier, capillary cells don't have to recover so much lost outer membrane receptor or mitochondrial volumes. The pace and how comprehensive the capillary cell recovery is will determine how well the interstitial space will revert back to optimal homeostasis.

Cutting off chronic interstitial space inflammatory fuel keys the capillary cell returns of the pivot and swing dance. When they dance, not only breach elimination more likely and interstitial space sanitation preserved at the expense of chronic inflammation, but it also unleashes the stemming and pacing of infrastructure refurbishment to itself and its allies as it nurtures end organ function. It does so through the reestablishment of its powerful feedback loop signaling system, involving its outer membranes and mitochondria, which had been disrupted by chronic inflammation.

The endothelial and capillary cell connection of shifting their outer membrane permeability to either energy or nitric oxide mitochondrial combustion keys their pluripotent purpose of *sanitizing* the interstitial space and *nurturing* the end organ while also *stemming* refurbishment to itself and interstitial space allies. A robust capillary cell dance becomes the foundation for wellness; age reversal if you will.

There are at least three variables to the equation of eliminating vascular inflammatory free radicals within interstitial spaces. They are as follows:

- The volume and diversity of free radical impingement.
- The health of the endothelial and capillary cell.
- The specificity and focus of arriving immune arsenal.

Any of these can lead to chronic inflammation but the one that affects the other two is free radical impingement. If vascular inflammatory free radical dispersion is overwhelming into the interstitial space it will cause capillaries to stop dancing and lead to a less competent immune arsenal entering the interstitial space. *Trafficking* goes into the mechanics of how vascular inflammatory free radicals block the capillary cell dance, disrupt feedback loops control of the interstitial to enable and increasing rogue immune arsenal passage into the interstitial space. How immune arsenal are trafficked into the interstitial space makes or breaks who controls the space.

Tackling chronic inflammation early and head-on does not require a lot of out of pocket money but rather a different mindset about lifestyle choice. It is the day to day practice of making good choices that blocks chronic inflammatory influences, keeps capillary cells dancing and nurtures wellness. Adjustments may not be easy, especially when it comes to addictions to drugs, sugar and nicotine. Implied here is the right to fail, but also to try again with the added help of family, friends and colleagues. Not only does it take a village but also motivation to be reeducated and disciplined about good habits, reading labels, as well as reading between the lines. When it comes to food, what sugar and fat grams actually mean requires heightened awareness of what is not revealed.

When addictions cause life's circumstances to go against us, it becomes easy to blame others. As victims we see our circumstances as being caused by outside influences. What is most important if we gain success over addictions is that we take personal; responsibility for them. Blaming others gives us ammunition to feel sorry for ourselves and continue the addiction.

Does chronic inflammation start with the expression from bad genes? Are we programed to fail? The accumulating evidence suggests that while our genes can make up us susceptible to alcohol or drug addiction, obesity, diabetes or elevated LDL cholesterol, lifestyle choices can trump these risks. If we adjust lifestyle early enough and stay at it, genetic risks don't have to play out. By aborting proinflammatory behaviors we provide momentum to stream healthier choices that can overcome our genetic profiles. Lifestyle can *frame wellness* regardless of our genetic risks.

No one escapes death but we can have input into longevity and the quality of that life extension. *Trafficking* details the mechanics of how capillary cells manage immune competence and what that means in avoiding age and disease related baggage.

-Robert L Buckingham, MD, FACP

CHAPTER 1

THE PARABLE OF THE FARMER

In a far- away land lived a gifted corn farmer. From season to season, no matter what, his sweet corn tasted better than anyone else.

Although no one could quite figure out why, he planted and sowed each year just like a regular. Each year, the plant and sow changed up slightly based on what the farmer called "prevailing conditions". This could mean how *cold* and how much *moisture* was in the soil. He never let a fall pass without mulching and tilling and would let fields lay bare for a season. No two years were alike. Other farmers would emulate but their corn did not quite stack up.

One year, things changed-*dramatically*. Beetles darkened the sky from the south. Their wing flap could be heard for miles away as they eclipsed the sun. Their intention was to eat anything green, which included corn.

Sensing the urgency to counter the beetles, the farmer amassed a team of specialists. Without much delay they presented their findings. Without swift intervention, nothing would be left of his corn crop.

At great expense large mesh nets were sown together and hoisted over some of the corn acreage. In another section, smelly manure was shoveled into the soil, and in still another cornfield, the immature stalks were drenched in water irrigation. The idea was to make the corn either less available or less appealing.

The nets, manure, and water did not work. The beetles savaged the corn crop. Within a few days only barren corn stalks remained. There was finger pointing, but the cause of failure was clear. No one recommended killing the swarming beetles.

Without any crop and the farmer now penniless, he could only walk away from the farm.

Can you translate the parable?

Robert L Buckingham, MD, FACP

The farmer represents a *capillary cell*, the soil, corn stalk and leaves the *interstitial space*, and the corn ear is the *end organ*. *The* beetle symbolizes the bombardment of *vascular inflammatory free radicals*. The netting, manure and water symbolize different types of *immune arsenal* meant to neutralize the free radicals. The consultants represent mesenchymal cells *and* the expense for their involvement is represented as capillary cell *energy combustion.*

Just as the horde of beetles destroyed the corn fruit, an overabundant and aggressive contingent of vascular inflammatory free radicals can bias chronic interstitial space inflammation and eventually destroy the end organ. In the parable, the mesh, manure and water are ineffective in limiting the beetle infestation. Within the interstitial space the inability to deliver enough T helper (killer) lymphocytes or monocytes will limit the capacity to eliminate inflammatory free radicals. Once the cash reserves are spent and the corn crop is ruined, the farmer walks away. Once the capillary mitochondria diminish in numbers to where they can no longer deliver energy to the capillary cell outer membranes, the capillary cell becomes incapable of interstitial space management and the end organ dies.

Could the outcome have been different? Yes, but the farmer would have had to change tactics and confront the beetle directly. The same is true with how capillary cells manage vascular inflammatory free radicals. In this case combining a lifestyle that diminishes the volume of free radicals penetrating the interstitial space coupled with the addition of immune arsenal that eliminates the free radicals would secure a different outcome.

CHAPTER 2

THE TRAP DOOR TO OUR IMMUNE SYSTEM

At the heart of immune operations are the endothelia of the vasculature system. Although all endothelia are codependent and contribute to optimal immune management, it is the capillary cell that facilitates the structured trafficking of immune arsenal combatants into interstitial spaces that secures an optimal working environment for end organs. What makes this job challenging is the volume and diversity of input that capillary cell outer membranes must integrate to enable effective interstitial space homeostasis. This becomes a constant moving target due to fluxes in end organ functional requirements, ever changing signals from other end organs, and the challenges of optimizing the interstitial space working environment. Even small missteps can chain react interstitial space compromise that will eventually limit capillary cell effectiveness and lead to a compromised end organ. At the heart of this compromise is the inability of capillary cells to deliver the right type or volume of immune arsenal into the interstitial space to maintain its sanitation. As sanitation deteriorates, end organ function declines. The end result is the tipping of the interstitial space towards chronic inflammation. When this happens, the space gets overrun by alternative sets of feedback loops from darker influences that divide the relationship between capillary and end organ cell. Nothing good comes from this divorce.

The remarkable part to the capillary cell's evolution is how its outer membranes have coupled with mitochondria to affect a dual purpose. On the one hand increased outer membrane permeability and mitochondrial energy combustion increase immune trafficking into interstitial spaces to eliminate inflammatory breach to restore homeostasis. On the other hand, decreasing outer membrane permeability and swinging mitochondrial combustion to nitric oxide engineers a restoration of its infrastructure, while increasing blood flow to enhance end organ functional capacity. In this manner changes in capillary cell outer membrane permeability adjustments coupled to mitochondrial combustion protects the interstitial space while also serving the end organ capacity to function. Capillary cell outer membrane permeability is tweaked based on what the end organ does and what kind of help it gets from interstitial space mesenchymal cells.

For their discovery it has been thought that capillaries were passive cells that had no meaningful input to management of the interstitial space. It was the end organ or the immune arsenal that did the regulating. Their purpose was to conduit gas exchange and energy substrate transfer to the end organ and enable immune arsenal entrance into the interstitial space when resourced by cytokines, white blood or mesenchymal cells.

This thinking has been turned inside out in the past two plus decades. Not only is the capillary cell far from a passive bystander, but a dynamic contributor to the interstitial space and end organ. Further, its success is linked to how well its outer membranes and mitochondria feedback loop each other, or how well they *dance. This dance* makes the interstitial space *harmonize* and the end organ *sing. The pivot and swing melody* reinforces optimal interstitial space *sanitation* and end organ *function.* It is connected to the *quality assurance* of ongoing capillary cell operations *as* well as to its allies-the mesenchymal cells and end organ itself. It turns out that the capillary cell is the head wagging the end organ tail.

It is the capillary cell dance rather than the end organ, mesenchymal cell or immune arsenal that enables the precise choreography of an immune response into the interstitial space to remove inflammatory breach and restore space homeostasis. The effectiveness of this choreography in eliminating inflammatory breach determines how clean the interstitial space remains, which portends how well the space will support the capillary-end organ cell relationship. It also forms the basis for how well the capillary cell will dance. If the interstitial space is perpetually clouded with inflammatory debris, capillary cells don't pivot and swing, as they get stuck in trying to eliminate this debris at the expense of their own restoration and end organ function. The persistence of interstitial space inflammatory debris blocks their dance. The imbalance cascades of host of capillary cell changes that render increasing dysfunction, which ties directly with associated declines in interstitial space hygiene and end organ ineptness. End organ disease venues, fatigue, pain and aging tag along. If inflammatory breach cannot be removed from the interstitial space, the capillary cell dance is blocked and this chain reacts the birthing of chronic inflammation. In this fashion capillary cells have become the *gatekeepers* the interstitial space homeostasis, the facilitators to the end organ function, and the stemming and pacing of rejuvenation to themselves and their mesenchymal and end organ cell allies.

The Capillary Cell Dance

The capacity for capillary cells to dual purpose is dependent on a robust pivot and swing dance based on feedback loop signaling exchanges between their outer membranes and mitochondria. Rigorous back and forth fluxing of outer membrane permeability means that capillary cells are busy receiving and sending myriads of different messages from a host of different contacts. It also means that they have been effective in trafficking immune arsenal into and out of their interstitial spaces to eliminate inflammatory breach and preserve its sanitation. It also implies that vascular inflammatory free radicals entering the interstitial space have been eliminated to enable the capillary outer membrane pivot of permeability. Finally, it means that capillary cell mitochondria have been guided through feedback loop signaling form outer membranes to shift combustion from energy to nitric oxide. The capillary cell dance forms the basis for wellness as it implies the stalling out of chronic inflammatory influences.

The extent to which endothelia don't pivot and swing, signals a capillary cell fail, and correlates with diminished mitochondrial volumes and outer membrane receptors. Chronic inflammation has established a permanent residence within the interstitial space and with it darker overtures to the fortunes of the end organ. Without the capillary cell dance, the interstitial space becomes dark and foreboding as the end organ becomes isolated and ineffective.

The Mitochondrial Combustion Swing

When capillary cell mitochondrial combustion swings to nitric oxide, three critically important adjustments occur to the capillary cell. First, within mitochondria, nitric oxide combustion *shifts acetyl coenzyme A* away from the energy producing cytochromes and Krebs cycle and instead is mobilized outside of the mitochondria towards ribosomes and rough endoplasmic reticulum. The shift in acetyl coenzyme A signals initiation of protein synthesis to replace worn out infrastructure. The shuttling of acetyl coenzyme A towards ribosomes in the cytoplasm is a necessary transition for capillary cell renewal and future quality assurance; in essence a prerequisite to disease prevention anti-aging. When acetyl coenzyme A migrates to ribosomes and rough endoplasmic reticulum it provides a usable energy substrate for protein synthesis. With uneven, insufficient or blocked nitric oxide combustion, acetyl CoA mobilization is ineffective thereby cascading protein replacement mistakes or inadequate protein repair.

Second, when mitochondrial combustion swings away from energy combustion, the outer membranes no longer require ATP for active transport of immune arsenal. The unused and accumulating cytoplasmic ATP, along with calcium ions, becomes an important signaling loop that feeds back to the mitochondrial matrix to halt energy combustion and activate the enzyme *nitric oxide synthetase* (NOS). NOS, not only increases nitric oxide production, but feeds back to the mitochondrial inner membrane cytochromes to inhibit the transfer of electrons. This serves as further impetus to block mitochondrial energy production. In this manner nitric oxide synthetase facilitates *nitric oxide production while simultaneously switching off energy combustion.*

Third, nitric oxide (NO) combustion results in the production of a diffusible gas. This gas can easily diffuse out of the mitochondria to activate protein synthesis, initiate replication and relax downstream arteriole smooth muscle to increase blood flow towards the affected capillary cell and its end organ partner. More blood flow means more oxygen and nutrient delivery to the capillary bed which in turn is transferred directly to the end organ. More oxygen and nutrient to the end organ translates into improved potential to function and implies that their mitochondria can rev energy combustion. As capillary mitochondria shift to nitric oxide combustion, end organ mitochondria alternatively shift to energy combustion to improve performance. When capillaries are dealing with interstitial space inflammatory debris, they shift to energy combustion and their end organ mitochondrial partners to nitric oxide production. The persistence of combustion in any one direction will eventually doom both the capillary and end organ cell due to the buildup of toxic free radical exhaust (superoxide or hydroxynitriles) from a one- sided combustion.

By blocking immune arsenal movement into the interstitial space, increasing blood flow to augment end organ function, stemming the refurbishment of its infrastructure and interstitial space allies, while diversifying combustion exhaust, capillary cell mitochondrial nitric oxide combustion *keys* capillary cell quality assurance and execution of optimal end organ function. The conversion to nitric oxide combustion does not happen *unless* capillary cell outer membrane permeability can downshift. The downshift is made possible by making the removal of vascular inflammatory free radicals and other inflammatory debris within the interstitial space as easy as possible. Lifestyle, lifestyle, lifestyle.

The inability to remove inflammatory breach within the interstitial space becomes the lynchpin of the capillary cell dance. In simple terms it becomes dependent on vascular inflammatory free radical impingement. In other words, the fluxing pivot and swing capillary cell dance becomes the *key facilitator* to blocking chronic interstitial space inflammation, and vascular inflammatory free radical impingements becomes the facilitator to block the capillary cell dance to enable a chronic inflammatory interstitial space beachhead. The health of the capillary cell dance becomes the quintessential basis for anti-aging mechanics.

The Chronic Inflammatory Coupe

The interstitial spaces of end organs can be described as a fluxing life bed of forces that either block or promote inflammation, and as a corollary, enhance or diminish the end organ. Impingement of the interstitial space by vascular inflammatory free radicals form the front lines of proinflammatory seeding and serve as fuel in the progression of chronic inflammation (Graph-3, appendix). Free radicals within interstitial spaces attach to membrane surfaces including endothelial and capillary cell basement membranes. Given enough attachment and subsequent pluming of immune arsenal towards them, they eventually disrupt the capillary cell dance by keeping capillary and endothelial cell mitochondria stuck in energy combustion. The sticking of combustion cascades a series of bad endothelial outcomes that include pseudocapillarization of their outer membranes, reduction of mitochondrial volumes and the further escalation of immune arsenal outliers into the interstitial space.

Chronic inflammation finds these immune arsenal vagabonds good for business and will utilize them to develop their own alternative feedback loop signaling system which will eventually supersede those of the failing capillary cell. This process of acquiring an alternative feedback loop signaling system defines the second stage of chronic inflammation and is known as the inflammatory matrix (Graph 3, appendix). The matrix expands operations by utilizing vascular inflammatory free radicals as fuel and outlier immune arsenal as an alternative feedback loop bridge to sway a proinflammatory interstitial space agenda. This alternative feedback loops coupled with abundant vascular inflammatory free radicals will further disrupt and disable capillary and endothelial cell outer membranes and block mitochondrial combustion of nitric oxide to eventually make endothelia a shell of what they once were. At this stage, capillary cells have become prepared for the final stage of chronic inflammation.

As outlier immune arsenal become preeminent the alternative feedback loops they create push mesenchymal cells to switch allegiance from capillary cells to chronic inflammation and those of the inflammatory matrix. Momentum clearly favors disruption of interstitial space homeostasis and isolation of the end organ as capillary cell function disintegrates. The coupe of the interstitial space has been successful, as endothelial and capillary cell mitochondrial volumes shrink, and outer membranes pseudocapillarize. The capacity to manipulate the interstitial space is now at a premium and this welcomes the emergence of the *chronic inflammatory anti-organ* (graph 3, appendix).

With free reign of capillary cell outer membranes, the anti-organ has the capability of implementing disease venues. With anti-organ emergence, rogue immune arsenal and mesenchymal cells can be parlayed into enabling bacteria, viruses, cancer cells, autoimmune complexes, thrombosis and scar tissue formation within the interstitial space. Along with vascular inflammatory free radical fuel, the anti-organ's alternative feedback loop system is now being utilized to initiate disease venues that not only isolate the end organ from the capillary cell but torture it as well. As disease venues mature, oxygen and nutrient are competitively utilized for infectious and cancer spread and for the development of the anti-organ at the expense of the true end organ.

Capillary Cell Outer Membranes: The Dance Leaders

Capillary cell outer membranes dance with mitochondrial combustion by fluxing their permeability. In this way their permeability adjustments lead as mitochondrial combustion follows their signal to increase or decrease energy or nitric oxide production. When outer membranes adjust permeability they modify outer membrane architecture, receptor exposures, electric voltage gradients, and pore size and density among others to increase or decrease resistance of immune arsenal entry into the interstitial space. It ends up being an elaborate symphony of sequenced movement that in the end requires energy to execute active transport of certain immune elements. As they flux permeability back and forth they are also telling mitochondria to adjust production of energy or nitric oxide to accommodate shifts in capillary cell purpose.

Their fluxing rigor, coupled with ample mitochondrial combustion of either energy or nitric oxide, facilitates optimal interstitial space homeostasis which then creates an optimal nurturing environment for the end organ to interact with the capillary cell. It also means that the interstitial space become much more difficult for vascular inflammatory free radicals to find chronic footing. As capillary cell outer membranes flux they execute dual functions that also support their own rejuvenation as well as that of its interstitial space allies. Fluxing not only adjusts immune arsenal trafficking, but also, through regional adjustments in blood flow caused by nitric oxide, will also increase oxygen and nutrient availability to the end organ.

Capillary cell outer basement membranes, particularly their basement membranes, have adopted different morphologies to accommodate different end organ functional requirements. For example, in the liver sinusoid, capillary cell basement membranes facilitate the mobilization of large volumes of industrial nutrient into the interstitial *space of Disse*, where it is collected by awaiting hepatocytes where it is processed into glycogen, and a complex array of different glycol and lipoproteins, enzymes, cholesterols, clotting factors, glucose and fatty acids. At the same time hepatocytes will decompose toxic waste through catabolizing different proteins, carbohydrates, fats and other toxic constituents.

Because hepatocytes have so much industrial machinery, they require capillary cells bring as much blood plasma constituent as possible to their outer membranes. Capillary cell basement membranes accommodate this hepatocyte request by loosening the regulation of plasma constituents entering the interstitial space. By acting more like a *sieve* than a *filter* or *barrier,* capillary cell basement membranes have biased lower voltage gradients, and are much more porous, with holes, gaps and slits within its infrastructure. This rapid and direct access of portal blood plasma to liver hepatocytes gives them greater access to industrial nutrient but comes with an increasing risk of potential exposures to circulating bacteria, viruses or cancer cells, which can also penetrate capillary cell outer membranes. The liver becomes a common portal of entry for the metastatic spread of cancer or the seeding of bacterial abscesses and viral infections.

In contrast to liver sinusoids, capillary cells that compose the *blood brain barrier* serve as barriers to any blood plasma constituent entering the cerebrospinal fluid (CSF), which bathes and provides nutrient and oxygen to the delicate brain cells. Capillary cells have very tight gap junctions with narrow tightly controlled channels and the basement membranes have no holes, gaps or slits. Together, with the capillary cell glycocalyx and continuous outer membrane, these outer membranes fend off most blood plasma constituents from entering the cerebrospinal fluid. Control of blood plasma entry by capillary cells is further instituted by energy driven *exocytosis,* as unwanted molecules are packaged within their cytoplasm and pushed back into the blood plasma. The control of unwanted blood plasma constituents into the cerebrospinal fluid is further refined by specialized mesenchymal cells known as *glial- astrocytes and pericytes.*

Deep within the brain groups of specialized capillary cells have formed the *choroid plexus.* In contrast to other capillary cells composing the blood brain barrier, capillary cells within the choroid plexus manufacture (*secrete*) cerebrospinal fluid. The blood brain barrier not only limits what gets into the cerebrospinal fluid, but through the combustion of nitric oxide, assists in shifting regional blood flow within the brain to accommodate adjustments in different brain activities.

Regardless of how capillary basement membranes have been modified to accommodate different end organ function, all capillary cells respond in kind when there is interstitial space breach. This means that choreographed trafficking of immune arsenal, into and out of interstitial spaces, follows similar signals and procedures regardless of which interstitial space is breached. For successful choreography the capillary cell outer membranes and mitochondrial must be pivoting and swinging.

Key to capillary cell choreography of trafficked immune arsenal is not just the energy they receive from mitochondria but their highly specialized outer membrane receptor network. This elaborate display of receptors and switches, when messaged, shift membrane infrastructure to expose different adhesion receptors (CAMS) which then attach specific immune arsenal within the blood plasma. These CAM attachments trigger a series of membrane changes that push these attached white blood cells into the gap junction or elsewhere for transit into the interstitial space. Decisions about what CAM to expose are based on a variety of signaling input from interstitial space immune arsenal, cytokines and mesenchymal cells at the breach staging area. Coupled with mitochondrial energy support, the capacity of capillary cell outer membranes to receive and send messages and the availability of different CAMs to attach selected immune arsenal for trafficking purposes increases the likelihood of breach removal.

In the manner the capillary cell actually supports *two end organs*, their true end organ, such as the brain, heart, kidney, lung, or liver, *and the immune system* end organ, which is used to pressure wash and sanitize interstitial spaces. All of this comes undone when chronic inflammation sets up shop within the interstitial space and blocks the capillary cell dance. This occurs, not just because of chronic festering of vascular inflammatory free radical fuel harbored within interstitial spaces, but the increasing penetration of the space by vagabond immune arsenal, that have no intention of participating in inflammatory breach removal. It is this group that sets up the alternative feedback loop messaging system within the interstitial space that eventually takes out capillary cell control. The sequence of excessive capillary cell mitochondrial energy combustion, superoxide overexposures, reduced mitochondrial volumes and pseudocapillarization of outer membranes repeats itself in nearly all interstitial spaces of all end organs as the same free radicals due the same collateral damage in all of them.

Capillary Cell Outer Membrane Fluxing Paces Interstitial Space Homeostasis

The fluxing of capillary cell outer membrane permeability, and the reverberating feedback loop signals that it sends to its mitochondria and interstitial space allies, sustains interstitial space homeostasis, increases oxygen and nutrient delivery to the end organ, prevents buildup of toxic free radical mitochondrial exhaust, and enables rejuvenation of its infrastructure as well as that of its allies. All of this while also applying the hammer in preventing the propagation of chronic inflammation. This makes capillary and endothelial cell outer membrane flux the *captain* of immune arsenal entry into the interstitial space and the viability of the end organ it serves. The key to maintaining captain status is minimizing interstitial space vascular inflammatory free radical impingement to a level where they can be successfully eliminated.

Thus capillary and endothelial outer membrane fluxing of immune arsenal trafficking into interstitial spaces becomes the weapon of wellness, disease prevention, end organ longevity and antiaging. Capillary cell outer membrane fluxing induces a feedback loop driven rejuvenation of its infrastructure and all intracellular organelles including mitochondria. This *mother of all feedback loops* also paces similar regenerative overtures to its interstitial space allies (mesenchymal cells) and end organ cells.

The hinge to outer membrane fluxing is its direct effect on shifting mitochondrial combustion. The subsequent switch to nitric oxide combustion keys regeneration but is the first to go when capillary cell outer membrane fluxing is prevented by chronic interstitial space inflammation. Shifting mitochondrial combustion to nitric oxide enables protein synthesis, which benchmarks regeneration of outer membrane receptors and cell infrastructure. Nitric oxide combustion becomes the key to capillary cell quality assurance and enables the cell to continue a rigorous outer membrane flux. Thus fluxing permeability not only sanitizes the interstitial space but also enables repair and replacement of capillary cell infrastructure so that the cell can continue optimal performance. This capillary cell fluxing feedback loops momentum transitions to include the outer membranes and infrastructure of its interstitial space allies.

When capillary cell outer membranes flux, mitochondria swing combustion thereby nullifying the buildup of toxic free radical exhaust (ROS-reactive oxygen species) caused by just one type of combustion. Excessive mitochondrial combustion of either nitric oxide or energy will cause the buildup of free radical exhaust (ROS) due to overutilization of exhausted antioxidants. Fluxing outer membrane permeability and shifting mitochondrial combustion back and forth enables antioxidants to be refurbished thereby nullifying infrastructure damage from accumulating free radical exhaust. This damage is particularly troublesome to mitochondrial and nuclear DNA. Once crosslinked, coding for protein synthesis becomes either silenced or defective, which further marginalizes capillary cell function.

Once affected by free radical impingement, capillary cell outer membranes flux permeability towards a choreographed immune arsenal response, which is driven by reductions in *cAMP (cyclic adenosine monophosphate)* and the switching on of membrane protein and tyrosine kinase enzymes. When activated, they cascade a series of membrane chain reactions that induce outer membrane infrastructure to bend and twist. The twisting exposes specific adhesion receptors that enable attachment of white blood cells, cytokines and other immune arsenal as they arrive from blood plasma. Once attached, white blood cells for example, can be rolled by other group of receptors (selectins) to a widened gap junction orifice where they are then suctioned into the gap junction channel. Once in the channel they are further sorted into regimens by other enzymes and receptors before they proceed to the interstitial space staging area.

Some immune arsenal forgo the gap unction channel and instead, after attachment to capillary cell outer membranes, are engulfed by *vesicles (endocytosis)* or pushed into trans-cellular *transport channels* which escort them to the interstitial space staging area. While this is occurring, capillary cell outer membrane switches are busy reducing membrane voltage gradients, opening pores, budding vesicles and transport channels, readjusting glycocalyx and basement membrane thickness, and widening gap junction orifices and channels. These adjustments are choreographed by capillary cells to introduce a precise immune arsenal response into the interstitial space to remove an inflammatory breach. When successful it creates the capillary cell pivot and swing dance as capillary cells reverse their permeability to cause a swing in mitochondrial combustion.

Execution of an effective immune arsenal response is based primarily on how much invader has arrived within the interstitial space and for how long they have been there. It is secondarily based on the *capacity* of arriving immune arsenal, the *density and diversity* of the capillary cell outer membrane receptors to successfully choreograph, and the *volume* of capillary cell mitochondria, which deliver the necessary energy surges that are required to transport some of the immune arsenal to the staging area. What becomes obvious based on previous discussions is that persistent free radical invaders will eventually disrupt the capacity of capillary cell outer membranes and mitochondria to accomplish their function. With any or all of these encumbrances the capillary cell dance gets blocked and chronic inflammation establishes a beachhead within the interstitial space.

When Capillary Cells Go from Oval to Flat

When capillary cells pivot and swing dance outer membrane configuration switches back and forth from *oval to flat*. Oval configuration facilitates immune arsenal movement through gap junctions, while a flat configuration increases their basement membrane exposure to end organ cells. Going flat increases the capillary cells capacity to interact with the end organ, and is linked to increased nitric oxide combustion, which enables increases in blood flow, oxygen and nutrient delivery to the end organ.

The shift from oval to flat or visa -versa becomes a strong indicator of what type of business the capillary cell basement membrane is transacting. More basement membrane exposure to the end organ implies effective interstitial space sanitation and a better working environment with the end organ. Less basement membrane exposure to the end organ implies the need for interstitial space inflammatory clean-up. With chronic inflammation, the capillary cell is biased to spend most of its time in oval mode thereby limiting basement membrane exposures to the end organ, while also denying increases in oxygen and nutrient delivery regardless of what end organs are signaling or requiring. Instead capillary cells are stuck pushing more immune arsenal into an already bloated interstitial space. All of this proinflammatory momentum plays into chronic inflammation as it begins to consolidate feedback loop control of the interstitial space. In this proinflammatory setting, capillary cells stay oval no matter what the end organ signals.

With age and chronic interstitial space inflammation, capillary cell outer membranes are preoccupied being oval or partially oval. This not only limits end organ function but enables capillary cell feedback loop signaling mistakes to compound. As capillary cells lock down an oval configuration they are at the same time handing over the keys of interstitial space homeostasis to chronic inflammation. As the capillary cell dance fails, mitochondrial volumes deteriorate, and outer membranes pseudocapillarize thereby creating a proinflammatory avalanche.

In other words, chronic inflammation has caused a chain reaction beginning with the blocking of the capillary cell dance and the loss of its feedback loops signals, which culminates in the demise of the end organ and its outer membranes, mitochondrial volumes and infrastructure. Whereas capillary cell DNA is crosslinked by superoxide reactive oxygen species, in contrasting fashion the end organ's DNA is being damaged by nitric oxide driven hydroxynitriles.

When chronic inflammation is reversed by reducing vascular inflammatory free radical impingement (AGEs, LDL cholesterol, lipo(a) etc.) within interstitial spaces, it takes some time for the capillary cell dance to remerge as many chronic inflammatory feedback loops within the interstitial space must unwind and be replaced by those originating from the capillary cell. For this reason, the capillary cell outer membrane reconfiguration of oval to flat, to reestablish intimacy with the end organ outer membranes, takes time. Just how far the capillary cell can dance, regain its feedback loops, and transition its configuration, speaks volumes about how aging, pain and fatigue can be reversed.

Free Radical Interstitial Space Impingement: How Chronic Inflammation Makes its Case

Capillary cell and interstitial space homeostasis can be a very well- oiled machine based on the fluxing dynamics of its pivot and swing dance and the subsequent swath of feedback loops it generates the affect all aspects of the interstitial space. If the dance is disrupted, the feedback loop mojo associated with it also goes. This creates the opportunity for an alternative feedback loops system to take its place and the interstitial space and end organ are cast into a dark shadow. Chief among risks to the capillary cell dance fail is the persistent abundance of vascular inflammatory free radicals. As these free radicals slither, often undetected into interstitial spaces, they have an affinity for basement membrane attachment.

Once attached, they not only silence basement membrane receptors but they also become the calling card for immune arsenal to be signaled from blood plasma. It is the persistent expansion of immune arsenal, attempting to ward off the abundant and diverse group of vascular free radicals on basement membranes, that carries momentum towards chronic inflammation.

If the free radical menace is not eliminated, inflammation becomes chronic and expands. The push of immune arsenal into the interstitial space *smoke screens* chronic inflammatory intent, as free radical persistence strains the capillary cell capacity to continue a sequenced immune arsenal response. With enough pestering and festering, the immune arsenal and mesenchymal cell messaging within interstitial spaces back to the capillary cell outer membranes becomes convoluted and mistake prone. A choreographed immune arsenal entering the interstitial space gives way to a more random array of mistake prone white blood cells and cytokines that are vulnerable to work against rather than for the capillary cell and its allies. This immune trafficking pivot transitions chronic interstitial space inflammation to the inflammatory matrix.

As capillary cell outer membranes become increasingly unable to sequence immune arsenal trafficking, the signaling display that they receive and send to interstitial space white blood cells, platelets, clotting factors, immunoglobulins, mesenchymal and end organ cells become confusing and even deceptive. It is the breakdown of this capillary cell feedback loop signaling display, which enables the inflammatory matrix to pick up the slack and offer an alternative. Immune mistakes within the interstitial space create their own momentum, as white blood cells and the cytokines they secrete, increasingly carve out a darker agenda. This proinflammatory momentum does not work out well for the capillary cell or its allies.

The mechanics of free radical basement membrane impingement begins with a persistent surge of capillary cell mitochondrial energy combustion to harness more and more immune arsenal into the interstitial space. The signal for energy combustion blocks the capillary cell dance, as capillary cell outer membrane permeability must traffic more and more immune arsenal into the interstitial space resulting in less time for their mitochondria to combust the regenerative nitric oxide gas. This combustion divergence takes its collective toll on the capillary cell, the interstitial space, mesenchymal cells and end organ. With less time spent in regeneration from nitric oxide the capillary cell homeostasis is upset with the result being a collapse of outer membrane receptor replacement and mitochondrial combustion apparatus. Superoxide free radical impingement on nuclear and mitochondria DNA puts the finishing touches on a disabled and ineffective capillary cell. The capillary cell not only cannot muster feedback loop signals to its interstitial space partners, buts its disabled outer membranes can easily be pirated and used to bring in immune arsenal remnants that feed rather than limit free radicals and disease venues within the interstitial space.

When chronic inflammation has successfully blocked the capillary cell dance it gets a controlling grip on what comes and goes within the interstitial space. Opportunity for disease venues becomes pro bono.

The Three Stages of Chronic Inflammation

In ideal situations, interstitial space sanitation where the removal of vascular inflammatory free radical impingements and other waste contaminants from the end organ are removed enabling capillary cells to pivot permeability and swing combustion. When this doesn't occur, free radicals impinge and stick to basement membrane surfaces to secure enough of an immune arsenal response where they are not permanently removed. *Stage one* of chronic inflammation (see appendix graph 3) is where vascular inflammatory free radicals have established a basement membrane beachhead, and are not removed. Their presence pesters the capillary cell into biasing more permeability time trafficking immune arsenal into the interstitial space, thereby causing their mitochondria to spend more time combusting energy to support the active transport of trafficked immune arsenal. This imbalance changes the energy to nitric oxide combustion equation within mitochondria, with combustion biases limiting the capillary cell's capacity to regenerate its infrastructure, outer membranes and mitochondria. The proinflammatory spiral has begun, but at this stage can be reversed quickly by reducing vascular inflammatory free radicals and turning inflammatory momentum in the opposite direction.

If vascular inflammatory free radicals are not reduced and there is continued impingement within the interstitial space, chronic inflammation moves to *stage II* (see appendix graph 3). This stage features the decline of the capillary cell as its pivot and swing dance is blocked. As capillary cell mitochondrial volumes decrease and outer membranes pseudocapillarize, a different kind of immune arsenal arrives into the interstitial space that has not been earmarked to remove inflammatory breach. These vagabond and rebel cytokines and white blood cells stir up the inflammatory pot and create confusion about purpose within the interstitial space. As they increase in stature within the interstitial space their capacity to spread their own brand of feedback loop messages increases, as the capacity for capillary cells to do the same declines. When rogue immune arsenal wrestle feedback loop control of the interstitial space away from the disabled capillary cell network, stage II of chronic inflammation has fully matured. When this occurs, mesenchymal cells within the interstitial space are now surrounded by hostile signaling influences and succumb to them. The betrayal of the capillary cell is now complete as immune elements and mesenchymal cells are answering to a different feedback loop system. At this stage, chronic inflammation can still be reversed through aggressive reductions in vascular inflammatory free radicals, but the reversal will take time due to how much decline the capillary cell and its allies have accrued.

When capillary cells achieve zombie status, and their outer membranes have been pirated and controlled by an alternative and darker feedback loop system, chronic inflammation is now ready to enter stage 3 (see appendix, graph 3) known as the anti-organ stage. It is in this stage that chronic inflammation establishes itself as an alternative end organ within the interstitial space, replete with its own feedback loop system, defenses, and immune arsenal. Chief among its tasks is to establish different disease venues within the interstitial space based on unique vulnerabilities of the true end organ. The disease venues further solidify anti-organ control of the interstitial pace and are additive to each other. As they progress, the true end organ withers, from combinations of diminished oxygen, and support from the capillary and mesenchymal cell partners. Like the capillary cell, the end organ cells eviscerate from the inside out, as their mitochondria spend too much time in nitric oxide mode, thereby producing enough unmitigated cyanide- like exhaust to destroy its DNA. As disease venues proliferate, the end organ declines. Aging accelerates as waves of pain and fatigue tag along. At this stage one thing is certain, there will be some type of disease within interstitial spaces such as scarring, infections, cancer, thrombosis or autoimmune disease. These outcomes are often deadly and require disease treatment intervention to stem progression. Disease treatment is side effect prone and can create its own set of disease venues. Welcome to modern medicine, the medical industrial complex and the proliferation of different treatment strategies to combat escalating diseases and complications from treatment in a never ceasing chain reaction.

At this stage, reversing chronic inflammation often requires more help than just reducing vascular inflammatory free radicals. Treatment of hypertension, elevated LDL cholesterols, blood sugars and other proinflammatory markers will be required in addition to treating infections, cancers, autoimmune diseases and thrombosis. Reversal will take time, and may be incomplete, based on the amount of DNA damage the capillary cell and its partners have accrued from the combination of the chronic inflammatory onslaught and the sustained block of its dance.

Why Capillary Cell Outer Membranes are so Unique

There are no other human cells that have as much outer membrane receptor diversity as those of capillary cells. Utilizing the feedback loops and permeability dynamics of three distinct outer membranes, capillary cells can nuance a vast array of immune arsenal responses to a mosaic of different interstitial space breach. At the same time, when breach is eliminated, its outer membrane permeability can turn quickly to shift mitochondrial combustion to nitric oxide which then gooses end organ function by delivering more oxygen and nutrient to their mitochondria. It is this dance, which parlays the function of both the immune system and end organ, which separates endothelia from other cells.

Trafficking is nuanced, not only from distress signals within the interstitial space from immune arsenal and mesenchymal cells, but also from adjacent capillary cells, downstream endothelia and distant end organs. In this way, the management of interstitial spaces and end organs becomes like a giant CIA operative. Coded secrets are constantly being forwarded as signaling loops between the capillary cell and its allies. The end game is to keep disrupters (such as vascular inflammatory free radicals) from influencing the interstitial space dynamics. Doing so enhances and protects end organ function. The system breaks down when the forwarding signals between capillary cells and allies get intercepted and switched up to betray rather than eliminate the offending free radical, or in the case of a disease venue, a bacteria, virus or cancer cell.

Unique to endothelial and capillary cell trafficking is the texturing that occurs from the influences of three different membrane surfaces. All three membranes function independently but are also codependent on what each membrane does best. Each membrane surface has their own sets of infrastructural proteins, enzymes, protein receptors and on-off switches that nuance trafficking. Included in this capillary cell outer membrane superstructure is a *continuous outer membrane*, which insulates the capillary cell cytoplasm and organelles from the blood plasma and interstitial space. There is also an abluminal *basement membrane*, which is the capillary cell contact membrane to the end organ. On the luminal side there is the *glycocalyx*, which buffers capillary cell blood plasma contacts with the continuous outer membrane while lending added support to the trafficking of immune arsenal. Capillary cell continuous outer membranes come together with contiguous capillary cells to form the *gap junction* or gap junction orifice and channel. It could be argued that the gap junction behaves as a fourth outer membrane, since it has its own sets of receptors, switches, voltage gradients and membrane barriers.

Based on where they are located and which end organ they serve, capillary cell outer membranes have unique properties that include structural *thickness, infrastructure proteins, voltage gradients, gaps, slits, pores, receptors and diaphragms.*

All outer membranes work together to facilitate capillary cell intended purpose. It is the quality and quantity of its receptor network that is most responsible for effective immune arsenal choreography. Change ups in outer membrane receptors nullifies precision to immune arsenal trafficking. This occurs when capillary mitochondria are not permitted to swing combustion to nitric oxide.

When chronic inflammation does impact outer membrane receptor density, the capillary cell glycocayx thins as their basement membranes thickens. Outer membrane voltage gradients, pores and other filters are compromised to enable compilations of vagabond immune arsenal entrance into the interstitial space. Choreographed immune arsenal trafficking is exchanged for a random and unnecessary array of white blood cells, cytokines, immunoglobulins and platelets. This becomes the backdrop to the evisceration of the capillary cell from the inside out, the deterioration of the interstitial space, the progressive isolation and dysfunction of the end organ, and the eventual scarring, cancer, infections, autoimmune disease and thrombosis from anti-organ disease venues.

It Takes Two to Tango

Lying in close proximity to the capillary cell continuous outer membrane, are clusters of *mitochondria* (see figure 1, picture 2 below and captioned in the following paragraphs). Mitochondria for decades have always been known as energy producing organelles, but only recently has it been understood that their combustion can shift and is linked to important feedback loops that regulate different cellular purposes.

Mitochondria are composed of an *outer membrane, intermembrane space, a coiled and redundant appearing inner membrane and central matrix*. The matrix is where combustion occurs and is also where mitochondrial DNA is housed. In contrast to nuclear DNA, mitochondrial DNA is exposed to combustion free radicals and lacks the protective telomere cap to its chromosomes, making it particularly vulnerable to free radical cross linkage. This vulnerability becomes relevant when mitochondrial combustion gets stuck in either energy (capillary cell) or nitric oxide (end organ cell) as an excessive build- up of reactive oxygen species from either combustion will exhaust anti -oxidants capacity to neutralize them and accumulate within the matrix to eventually cross link DNA and render it useless. This becomes a major contributor to their suicide and loss of mitochondrial volumes within the cell.

Within the mitochondrial matrix is an elaborate combustion infrastructure, which includes the Krebs cycle and the mechanics of pyruvate and fatty acid energy substrate conversion to *acetyl CoA*. The production of acetyl CoA from energy substrate becomes the dominant hub to the swinging of mitochondrial combustion. Depending on whether mitochondria are combusting nitric oxide or energy, acetyl CoA will be mobilized either to ribosomes outside of the mitochondria for proteins synthesis or fed into the Krebs cycle within the mitochondrial matrix to generate hydrogen, which is then transported to the cytochromes to produce more energy.

Between the mitochondrial matrix and intermembrane space is the snake like inner membrane, which harbors a potent *voltage gradient* and is where the *cytochromes* are imbedded. Within the cytochromes electrons are transferred in a series of chain reactions that releases hydrogen into the intermembrane space to enhance its voltage gradient. As hydrogen accumulates, some of even most of it is eventually reintroduced back into the matrix at *cytochrome V* to assist the final step of energy production, the conversion of ADP to ATP, in the presence of *oxygen, phosphorus,* and *ATP synthase.* ATP becomes the predominant energy molecule within all cells and mitochondrial combustion is the method used by all end organs in obtaining the majority of its energy requirements.

Mitochondrial *combustion* means that *oxygen* is required, and when coupled with pyruvate or fatty acids, produces acetyl CoA and energy or nitric oxide. When oxygen is utilized for combustion purposes, it creates a free radical exhaust, which is known as *reactive oxygen species or ROS.* Both combustion of energy and nitric oxide produce their own type of toxic ROS. Toxic exhaust becomes a problem when mitochondria cannot swing combustion back and forth, such as when they get stuck combusting too much energy. This is best exemplified when capillary cell outer membranes persistently call out for more energy to mobilize immune arsenal into interstitial spaces. This occurs with chronic interstitial space inflammation, where capillary cell mitochondria are called out to continuously produce more energy. As they do, the produce more superoxide exhaust, which eventually depletes anti-oxidant reserves and destabilizes mitochondrial DNA.

As capillary cell mitochondrial DNA is denatured from excessive energy combustion, end organ cell mitochondria are stuck in the opposite direction- nitric oxide combustion. Their mitochondrial exhaust produces excessive quantities of *hydroxynitriles (cousins to cyanide), which can also deplete anti-oxidants and has a similar toxicity profile to DNA as superoxide.* This malignant DNA chain reaction, involving co linked capillary and end organ cell mitochondrial exhaust, is why it is so important for capillary outer membranes to flux permeability and dance mitochondrial combustion back and forth. By swinging mitochondrial combustion back and forth, exhaust end products become diversified and easier to neutralize by antioxidants before they damage DNA. In addition, as combustion swings and shuts down one type of combustion, antioxidants utilized for combustion exhaust that has been turned off have the chance to re accumulate, thereby further nullifying toxic ROS buildup.

Mitochondria DNA cannot sufficiently code for the replacement of all its matrix and inner membrane infrastructure. This means that for capillary cell mitochondria "to *replace, repair and replicate*" they also require nuclear DNA participation. Because of this DNA divestiture, that is unique to mitochondria, their capacity to initiate *fission, fusion,* replication or suicide is based on how well they are swinging their combustion. If they are swinging optimally, mitochondria fuse and replicate. If they are stuck in energy or nitric oxide combustion mode, toxic free radical exhaust builds up (ROS) and they go into fission and suicide mode. When this occurs, their volumes within the cell deteriorate.

This opens the door for the cell to cannibalize from the inside out, as lack of energy support from anemic mitochondria within the capillary cell, limits what and how much outer membranes can actively transport to the interstitial space. This chain- reacts a series of adverse events that hurts end organ function and escalates de sanitation of the interstitial space. With chronic interstitial space inflammation, capillary cell mitochondria overheat in energy combustion, increase superoxide exhaust, accelerate damage to their DNA, and decrease their volumes through combinations of suicide and fission. As they do, the capillary cell outer membranes throw the white flag and pseudocapillarize, thereby losing their capacity to choreograph immune arsenal entry into the interstitial space. With the build-up of an increasingly rogue immune arsenal within the interstitial space chronic inflammation now has the means to seize control of space battle ground by outsourcing a rogue and alternative sets of feedback loops that are meant to confuse and deceive. The deception is executed by vagabond and rebel white blood cells and cytokines which have entered the intestinal space by mistake. The interstitial space becomes dark and conducive to a number of different disease risks.

Capillary cell outer membranes and mitochondria are anatomically in close proximity for a reason. They mutually support each other's interests by responding in kind to each other's feedback loop signals., which is how and why they dance. Without chronic inflammation, they improve each other's function. Chronic interstitial space inflammation does the opposite, as it cannibalizes capillary cell mitochondria, which in turn precipitates a pseudocapillarization of its outer membranes.

The Mechanics of the Pivot and Swing Dance

As capillary cell outer membranes uptick permeability to increase immune arsenal trafficking, their outer membranes bend and twist to expose unique sets of receptors. These receptors or CAMS (adhesion molecules) then facilitate attachment of specific immune arsenal. As this occurs, capillary cell outer membranes send feedback loop signals for mitochondria to swing combustion to energy so that they will release calcium and energy to the outer membranes to support mobilization of immune arsenal. Capillary mitochondria become dependent on outer membranes to downshift permeability at some point so that they can shift combustion and refuel their antioxidants. This shift becomes dependent on satisfactory breach elimination within the interstitial space which in large part is based on how much proinflammatory free radical fuel is harbored there. If breach is eliminated, the capillary cell dance proceeds. If not it is blocked. To the degree it is blocked is to the degree that capillary cells will decline, as their mitochondria will spend too much effort combusting energy and not enough producing nitric oxide. A proinflammatory chain reaction proceeds from this point and can lead the capillary cell to purgatory. Everything else within the interstitial space and beyond will follow.

The feedback loops that capillary cell mitochondria respond to involve outer membrane calls for calcium ions and energy. When outer membrane permeability decreases, and active transport of immune arsenal is no longer required, calcium ions and energy (ATP) accumulate within the capillary cell's cytoplasm. This accumulation feeds back to nearby mitochondria to stop energy production and shift combustion to nitric oxide. When this occurs, calcium ions re accumulate within the mitochondrial matrix and adjacent smooth endoplasmic reticulum. The capillary cell shift to nitric oxide production induces a transcellular rejuvenation, with repair and replacement of worn out proteins, which include those of outer membrane receptors and within the mitochondrial matrix and inner membrane. With repair of mitochondria comes more fusion and replication which increases their volumes.

This built in auto-reset creates a capillary cell quality assurance enabling optimal performance in future inflammatory breach to the interstitial space. These powerful feedback loops, between outer membranes and mitochondria occurring within capillary cells, ripple through the interstitial space to include those of mesenchymal cells and the end organ. In this manner as capillary cells pivot and swing, their cellular allies will also be involved in adjusting outer membrane permeability and either increasing energy combustion or rejuvenating their infrastructure. The key is in the flux, spending too much time in either combustion will doom the cell.

The power of the capillary cell pivot and swing dance therefore becomes the basis for sustaining optimal interstitial space homeostasis and end organ function. Its outer membrane and mitochondrial pivot and swing will feedback loop with close by downstream arterioles. This helps to integrate purposes and keep each cell on the same functional page. The capillary cell pivot and swing dance paces a homeostasis rhythm involving the interstitial space, immune arsenal, end organ, interstitial space mesenchymal cells and downstream endothelia. This rhythm becomes the antidote to anti-aging, fatigue and pain, as it blocks chronic inflammation while facilitating its own and allied rejuvenation.

The more chronic inflammation is enabled to parlay influence within the interstitial space, the more likely that the capillary dance is compromised and the ripple effect of malaligned feedback loops through the interstitial space will occur.

Figure One

Picture 1

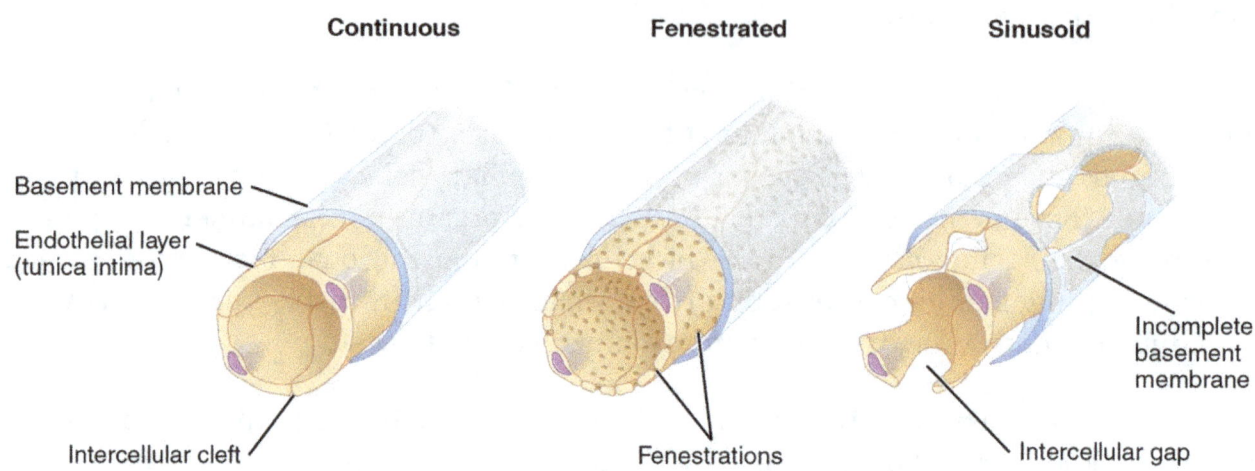

Continuous   **Fenestrated**   **Sinusoid**

Basement membrane

Endothelial layer
(tunica intima)

Intercellular cleft

Fenestrations

Incomplete
basement
membrane

Intercellular gap

Picture 2

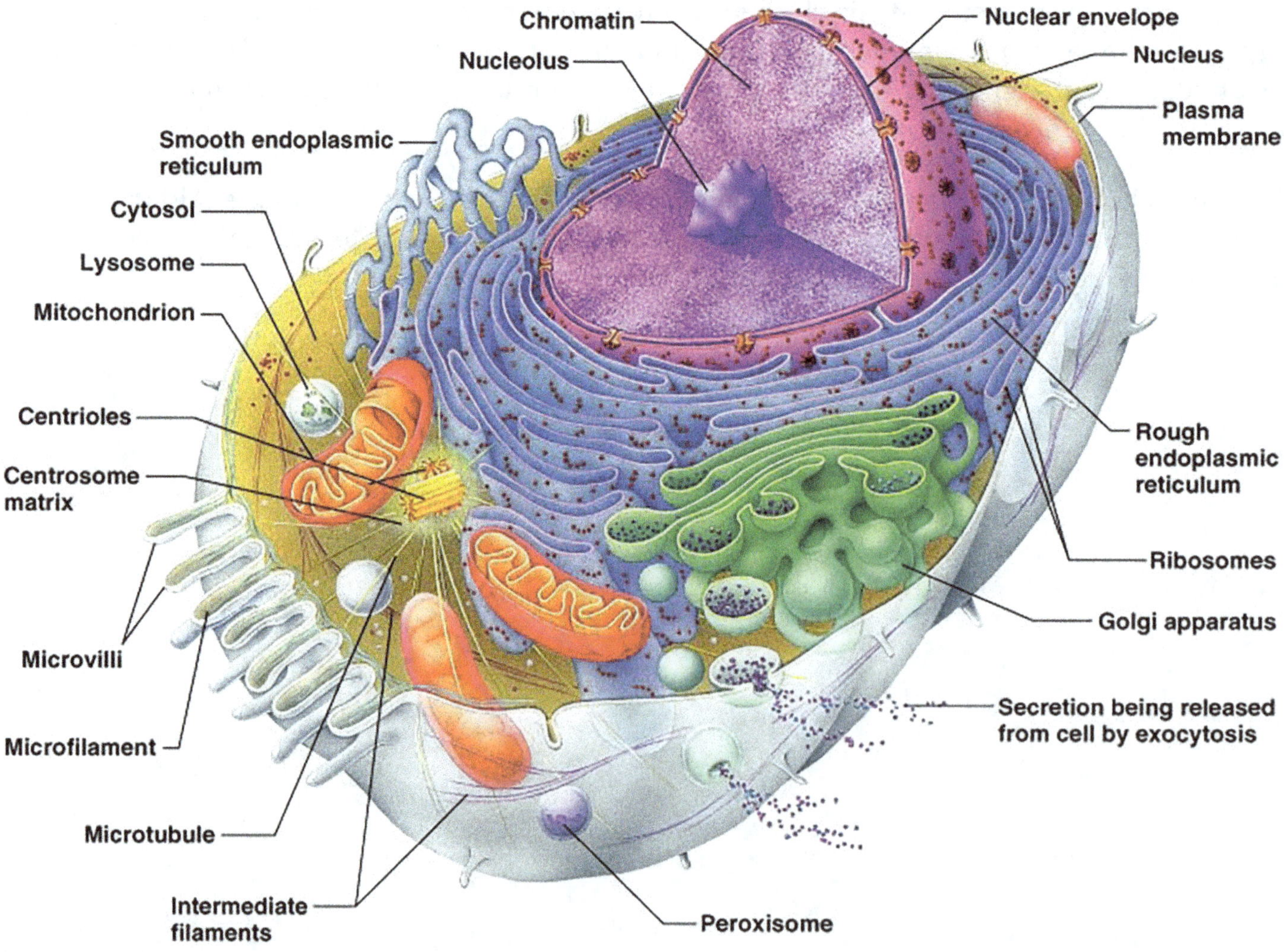

Chromatin

Nucleolus

Smooth endoplasmic
reticulum

Cytosol

Lysosome

Mitochondrion

Centrioles

Centrosome
matrix

Microvilli

Microfilament

Microtubule

Intermediate
filaments

Peroxisome

Nuclear envelope

Nucleus

Plasma
membrane

Rough
endoplasmic
reticulum

Ribosomes

Golgi apparatus

Secretion being released
from cell by exocytosis

In the above figure, picture 1 depicts different capillary cell basement membrane morphologies that range from a tightly knit group of endothelial cells seen in the blood brain barrier to a loosely arranged group of capillary cells with gaps that are seen in the liver sinusoid. It should be noted that both the basement membrane and the continuous outer membrane have evolved strategically to accommodate different end organ functions. As more gaps and fenestra emerge, the end organ will get exposed to more blood plasma constituents thereby increasing their risk of potential exposure to toxins, foreign invaders or other contaminants.

Picture 2 depicts a compilation of a 3-dimensional capillary cell. The mitochondria are identified as the orange sausage shaped structures with the coiled redundant appearing inner membrane. It is the inner membrane, which harbors a very potent voltage gradient, and is where the five chambered cytochromes of electron transfer are housed. It turns out the electron transfer through the cytochromes accomplishes two functions. First, by amassing hydrogen ions within the intermembrane space, it maintains the inner membrane voltage gradient. Second, by enabling the reintroduction of hydrogen ions back into the matrix at cytochrome V, the inner membrane facilitates the potential production of large volumes of energy. In the capillary cell, it is this energy surge that facilitates the active transport of immune arsenal into the interstitial space.

When capillary cell outer membranes down shift permeability and energy expansion is no longer necessary, calcium ions and ATP accumulate in the cytoplasm, easily penetrate the mitochondrial outer membrane, and eventually feedback loop the activation of the enzyme *nitric oxide synthase,* which induces production of nitric oxide. As is so often the case in biology an enzyme, like nitric oxide synthase, will activate one effect while blocking another. In this case as it activates nitric oxide production it simultaneously blocks the electron transfer of cytochromes thereby blocking energy combustion. This shift in mitochondrial combustion signals a shift in capillary cell purpose, away from interstitial space sanitation and towards renewal of its infrastructure while also increasing end organ capacity to function.

How the Capillary Cell Mitochondrial Matrix Multitasks

In figure 1, picture 2 above, note the proximity of the mitochondria to the voluminous *rough endoplasmic reticulum* and attached *ribosomes.* When capillary cell shift combustion to nitric oxide, these two organelles will take acetyl coenzyme A from the mitochondrial matrix and initiate protein synthesis for repair and replication purposes. When energy combustion gets reinitiated, nitric oxide synthase is shut down, ATP synthase is activated and acetyl coenzyme A gets shuttled into the Krebs cycle for purposes of making hydrogen ions for cytochrome electron transfer.

Also in picture two above, the close relationship between mitochondria and smooth endoplasmic reticulum is demonstrated. It is in the mitochondrial matrix and smooth endoplasmic reticulum where most of the cell's calcium ions are stored. When mitochondria are combusting energy, calcium ions are released and return when nitric oxide production occurs.

Another important mitochondrial matrix combustion outcome is the production of *heme* and antioxidants which include the *glutathione* and *manganese superoxide dismutase families*. Heme is a complex symmetric crown- like molecule, composed of a centrally charged iron. The heme molecule, with the exposed iron, is incorporated into the cytochromes to facilitate electron transfer. Heme production is complex, likely occurs during nitric oxide combustion, and requires a mosaic of precursors and enzymes found in the mitochondrial matrix, smooth endoplasmic reticulum and cytoplasm.

Other essential mitochondrial matrix feedback loops involve protein synthesis, repair and replication. In these instances, mitochondrial matrix DNA works in close conjunction with nuclear DNA to code for necessary protein replacement. This requires close communication with ribosomes, rough endoplasmic reticulum and *Golgi apparatus* (see Figure 1, picture 2).

The Nucleus and Nucleolus –The Keepers of the Code

All capillary cells have a single large *nucleus* (figure one above-picture 2). The nucleus contains *chromatin*, or DNA chromosomes which code for synthesis of most of the cells proteins, including some within their mitochondria. In contrast to mitochondrial DNA, nuclear chromosomal DNA is protected by a *telomere cap* which can rapidly shrink in the presence of chronic interstitial space inflammation. This is due to the blocked capillary cell dance and the subsequent deactivation of the enzyme *telomerase,* which regenerates the telomere cap.

Within each endothelial cell is one nucleus, and within the nucleus, a nucleolus. When activated by the nucleus, the nucleolus copies DNA to make *messenger RNA (mRNA)*. Accurate copying of DNA to mRNA is the second step to effective protein synthesis, as the copied DNA must not contain too many errors from free radical cross linkage. Once copied, mRNA travels to ribosomes located on or near rough endoplasmic reticulum (see above Figure-picture 2). The *translation* of mRNA into protein synthesis is facilitated by mitochondrial acetyl coenzyme A (acetyl CoA) arrival to ribosomes, as a result of the mitochondrial combustion swing to nitric oxide.

Small missteps within the DNA infrastructure itself, its *transcription* to mRNA or in translation to make proteins in ribosomes will induce silencing or malfunction of coded protein replacement. Inept proteins may be less capable than the worn out proteins they are replacing. In the case of capillary cell outer membrane protein receptors, malfunctioning protein replacement silences their capacity to attach immune arsenal which leads to pseudocapillarization. These mistakes which silence receptors cascade the leaking of more mistakes that perpetuate the vagabond immune arsenal constituency into interstitial spaces. Chain reactions of inappropriate immune arsenal responses into interstitial spaces can occur based on silenced or malfunctioning capillary cell outer membrane protein receptors.

Limiting nuclear DNA free radical cross linkage is dependent on the capillary cell dance and preventing the accumulation of superoxide ROS. As more DNA is damaged, it becomes harder for capillary cells to recover from the ravages of chronic inflammation. This means that even with great reductions in vascular inflammatory free radicals there will be holes of vulnerability within their outer membrane receptor network. This requires even further scrutiny to vascular inflammatory free radicals and perhaps medicinal intervention to prevent disease venue progression. It is the volume of DNA damage that determines whether capillary cells can effectively reverse course from chronic inflammation. There is a point of no reversibility. When it occurs, death is a preferable option rather than trying to slog through one disease venue after another.

The Supporting Cast

The word "other" implies less important, but when it comes to capillary cell operational homeostasis, all organelles are required as part of their feedback loop cross checking infrastructure. Whereas ribosomes manufacture proteins on the basis of messenger RNA input, the rough endoplasmic reticulum (rough ER) takes the finished proteins and provides "fit and finish", as it bends and twists the newly minted proteins into their finished dimensions. Once completed, the proteins are then stamped or certified for function by the *Golgi apparatus* (see figure 1 above, picture 2). Once certified, the proteins are distributed and integrated to where they belong.

The Golgi apparatus also "buds" *lysosomes*. Lysosomes are membrane enclosed *vacuoles* that decompose toxic fatty acids and intracellular fat soluble waste. As such they act as a lipid antioxidant to proinflammatory fatty acid free radicals. The decontamination process is known as *lipid peroxidation*. With aging and chronic inflammation, the capacity for the Golgi apparatus to bud lysosomes is diminished making it more likely that toxic fatty acids will roam the cell's cytoplasm and cause damage.

Not far from capillary cell mitochondria are *peroxisomes and smooth endoplasmic reticulum*. Peroxisomes facilitate shortening of longer fatty acid chains to 16 carbons or less by uncoupling carbon atoms. The shorter chained fatty acids can then be mobilized into the mitochondrial matrix where they can be further catabolized through *beta oxidation* to make usable substrate -*acetyl CoA, succinyl CoA or propionyl CoA*. In addition, peroxisomes can also facilitate bending fatty acids into usable forms so that they can be incorporated into membrane surfaces, as part of nitric oxide generated membrane repair or replacement.

The processes of lipid peroxidation that occurs in peroxisomes and lysosomes can go in either direction depending on the feedback loop signals they receive. In other words, these organelles can facilitate fatty acid breakdown into shorter carbon chains or their reconstruction into longer chained fatty acids. In this manner these organelles are part of larger metabolic feedback loop within the cell, that counterbalances pyruvate and fatty acid mitochondrial combustion, with cytoplasmic glycolysis and gluconeogenesis.

Whereas the rough endoplasmic reticulum (see figure 1 above, picture 2) is primarily involved with reshaping newly minted proteins, the *smooth endoplasmic reticulum* (smooth ER) facilitates calcium ion storage and regulating heme homeostasis. In the case of heme, the smooth ER recycles it by catabolizing older heme molecules into smaller and more usable intermediates. The smooth ER also sends fatty acid signaling messages to lysosomes and peroxisomes to increase or decrease the production or catabolism of longer chained fatty acids. In this manner, the smooth ER also plays an important role in regulating how much fatty acid is available for mitochondrial combustion of acetyl CoA. This becomes an important feedback loop tool is regulating pyruvate combustion and limiting insulin resistance.

In the big picture of which substrate is preferred for mitochondrial combustion, it is vital to see the interconnectedness of cytoplasmic gluconeogenesis, and glycolysis with lysosomes, peroxisomes and smooth endoplasmic reticulum. How they interact will be an important part of how well cell's limit insulin resistance or the buildup up of pyruvate necessitating its conversion to glucose by gluconeogenesis. With aging and a host of other regulatory biases, gluconeogenesis increases, thereby increasing blood sugars and predisposition to diabetes.

The Capillary Cell VEGF Dilemma

Sometimes capillary cells, are signaled to reproduce new capillaries to improve oxygen delivery to the end organ. The signal for capillary cells to replicate can be complex, as end organ demands for more oxygen are often clouded by chronic inflammatory influences within the interstitial space and by downstream large vessel obstructive plaque, which limits blood flow upstream, no matter how much capillaries try to do to increase it. This means that capillary replication to form new blood vessels will be futile, unless larger downstream vessels are either non obstructed or can provide collateral circulation utilizing other resources, to prop up additional downstream blood flow.

In cases where chronic inflammation has established alternative feedback loops, capillary cells are signaled to replicate to assist anti-organ disease venues. In these cases, the anti-organ *uses* the already compromised capillary cell for its own purposes to support cancer growth or populating the interstitial space with bacteria or virus. In this manner, capillary replication will cause further deterioration of the true end organ.

Replication signals for new capillaries to increase oxygen and nutrient delivery to the interstitial space can promote pro or anti-inflammatory agendas and depends on who is in control of the interstitial space. When the capillary cell is in control and replication signals are the result of increased end organ workload, such as skeletal or heart muscle being exercised, capillary replication if beneficial and supports optimal interstitial space homeostasis. When replication signals come from the anti-organ, through alternative feedback loops generated by rogue immune arsenal as a result of cancer of infectious spread, it will further compromise the interstitial space and reduce true end organ function. Where from whom the feedback loop originates is the catch 22 of *VEGF (also known as vascular endothelial growth factor)* or other growth factors. The where and from whom of VEGF dispersal will determine if capillary cells replication will work for the end organ or anti-organ.

When VEGF is capillary cell enabled, it induces *centrosomes* (see figure one above, picture 2) within the capillary cell's cytoplasm to disassemble the nuclear membrane and initiate replication of its DNA. This cascade eventually causes cell division (cell mitosis). Even with significant downstream large vessel obstructive plaque which limits blood flow, capillaries upstream will replicate anyway in hopes that larger vessels downstream will figure it out and find a way to bring more blood flow upstream. When the downstream answer is collateral circulation, blood flow increases by diverting it from other end organ regions that are not calling for more oxygen. The stakes of blood flow *addition by subtraction* can be high as blood taken away could cause its own sets of hypoxic-ischemic risks to the end organ. Unless downstream large vessel plaque is stabilized or reversed, upstream VEGF induced capillary cell replication becomes a band aide of slow end organ hypoxic torture. End organ cellular atrophy and interstitial space scarring often result. This result is typical of brain or heart outcomes, where dementia and heart failure linked to different types of interstitial space scarring commonly occur.

The Outer Membrane Three Ms

The capillary cell outer membranes also contain miniscule *microvilli, microtubules and microfilaments* (Figure one above-picture 2). Microvilli *act as small crypts (pockets), to* increase the surface area of the capillary cell continuous outer membrane, which enables further expansion of receptor surface area. Microfilaments contain fibrils of *actin and myosin*, which in the presence of released mitochondrial energy (ATP) and calcium ions, facilitate actin-myosin sliding. When actin-myosin fibrils slide, the filaments shorten (contract), thereby enabling a flat capillary cell to change configuration and become oval. The flat configuration facilitates basement membrane interaction with the end organ and occurs with capillary cell mitochondrial nitric oxide combustion. The oval configuration implies interstitial space inflammatory breach and biases mobilization of immune arsenal into the interstitial space. The oval configuration opens and widens the gap junction orifice and channel respectively thereby enabling a more rapid pace of immune arsenal mobilization.

The third member of the capillary cell outer membrane M family is the microtubules. The microtubules help facilitate capillary cell mitosis, as they connect the capillary cell continuous outer membrane to the *centriole/centrosome complex* (figure 1, picture 2). When capillary cells divide, the microtubules enable the splitting and re- splicing of the continuous outer membrane, as capillary cell infrastructure is replicated and divided into 2 cells.

The cross checked homeostasis of all the outer membrane apparatus is dependent on how well the capillary cells dance. Any proinflammatory momentum which biases a block of the capillary cell pivot and swing dance will cause chain reactions of adverse inflammatory ripples that will code for a darker feedback loop system.

CHAPTER 3

THE PARABLE OF THE OLD WOMAN

In a land far away, there lived an old woman. She was different from other old women because she did not conform to the customary way of doing things. Her habit was to take early morning walks into the woods, pick berries, leaves, and nuts, and then would use them to make daily teas, stews and soups. Every Friday she opened her patio to guests to casually sit and sample what she had prepared that day. Word go out about Friday afternoons at the old woman's patio and soon waiting lines formed for a chance to sit and sample.

Her soups were different from the rest in that they tasted so much better and the locals swore they felt better just with a single bowl. Owners of local eateries became jealous and started witchcraft rumors, although the taste of the soups trumped all of the hearsay.

What made matters worse, was how the old woman looked. Her complexion, for 60ish, was flawless. Her hair remained thick and long, and she walked quickly with her wispy legs gliding in stride with her torso. She kept an upright posture and appeared taller than most in part due to her upright stature. She greeted even strangers with a smile and never forgot a name after being introduced once. When cooking, cleaning or foraging, she could be heard singing or whistling.

Her soups and stews were only from ingredients gathered that day, which made them quite different from the usual eatery. The difference is not just in taste but how you felt afterwards. It was compared to taking medicine.

This did not go over well with the local eateries. When witchcraft rumors were ignored, they turned to the local magistrate. With greased palms, a deal was made to have her removed.

With a warrant in hand, the magistrate would pay a call on the old woman.

"Good morning. I am detective Hope. I have a warrant for your arrest for food poisoning and witchcraft."

The portly magistrate shoved the door open and began to search the premises for evidence. Not knowing what he was looking for, he fumbled through neatly sorted piles of leaves and berries as they spilled to the floor. The pantry cabinets were opened and left ajar with similar results. The old woman could only stand speechless and in dismay, shocked as the detective dismantled her kitchen.

Within minutes, and with everything either on the floor or disheveled, the old women's hands were tied and she was led out of her house and booked in the local jail for poison and witchcraft. It didn't matter that there was no evidence for either.

Years passed and the memories of her soups and teas faded and the eateries were doing business as usual. In jail, now for several years, the old woman had become frail and haggard. Barely able to walk she was released on her own recognizance. At this point she was so frail that most felt that death would be imminent. She limped back to her dilapidated cottage alone and penniless. She crumpled up into a corner, found a moth eaten old blanket and fell into a deep sleep. The next morning, she limped out of her cottage at the crack of dawn and took her first walk in years. She picked, whistled and sang. Afterwards she came home, dug up an old pot and wood, pumped some water from a nearby well and began stewing.

Within days she looked different. The limp went away, the gait lengthened and posture returned to upright. As her pace and temp returned to what it once was, so did her vitality, skin tone and hair texture. Little by little the cottage came back to life as bits and pieces of repair were accomplished.

Before she could begin her Friday afternoon socials, detective Hope would pay another visit to the old woman.

With an abrupt knock, the old woman opened the door. Detective Hope's stood there and stared at the old woman. He was caught off guard.

"You're not who I am looking for! Where is the old woman, and who are you?"

"I am she, as she started pouring hot soup into a bowl. Would you like some?"

"You're lying! Where is the old woman that was released from jail?"

"I am she. No one else lives here but me," as her piercing blue eyes caught up with his.

"I am not leaving until you bring her to me!" He sat down in front of the bowl of hot soup. The old woman handed him a spoon and he reluctantly partook. As he was eating, he looked her over again and said," rove to me that you are her!"

"Do you like my soup? Would you like another bowl?"

"This soup proves nothing, but yes, another bowl would be fine." He quickly finished it but was not amused.

"Come back tomorrow. I promise I'm not going anywhere. I will give you more proof."

"You have 24 hours. Don't waste my time." He left in a huff as he slammed the door shut.

The next day became the next day and the next day. Each time detective Hope would appear, ask questions, demand that old woman come out of hiding, and also eat the hot soup of the day. And each time the tone of the visits changed from being confrontational to more friendly. His original plan was to soften her up by applying pressure but the reverse was happening. He started looking forward to the visits. And something strange was happening. He began paying attention to his hair, teeth and boots.

After a few weeks, he knocked at the door with a hand full of just picked wild flowers.

"Uhh, can I call you Kate?" as the old woman took the flowers and promptly placed them in a wooden vase.

"Thank you for this beautiful bouquet. I am Kathryn, but you should know my name as you booked me previously as Kate".

"You... you, I mean.... really......uhh... are the same old woman? I mean...... you.... you really are her. How can it be so? You.... you look nothing like what I remember. Please don't take that the wrong way!"

"Let's go for a walk. Grab that sack behind you. With that she was out the door and walking on a narrow but well -worn path with the detective following close behind.

As the pace slowed Kate began filling the gunny sack with various leaves, berries and nuts. She simultaneously greeted squirrels, and said hello to rabbits and birds. When the sack was nearly full, they turned around and went back to the cottage.

More weeks passed but things were changing. The detective was falling out of his uniform. In addition, he was no longer limping. Terse grumpiness was replaced with softer tones belying empathy. Was he feeling .... love?

The detective sobered up to the truth. The old woman's concoctions were not poisoning but rather life giving. How could he have been so wrong?

Months passed, love grew and then wedding bells chimed. After the nuptials, the detective retired and became first assistant to Kate and her soup making. They opened the patio up full time to locals, who couldn't get enough of her freshly made soups. In spite of their "advanced age" the two as one found happiness together for decades.

Can you translate the parable?

In the parable, Kate the old woman is a capillary cell, the local eateries represent vascular inflammatory free radicals (inferior food) and rogue immune arsenal (deceit and false accusations). The detective is the mesenchymal cell and the locals symbolize the end organ. When the old woman was in her daily rhythm, she facilitated a superior soup, tea and stew (oxygen and nutrient) that was well received as nurturing to the locals (end organ).

As this enfolds, local eateries felt the impact of her "all natural and healing" concoctions and felt their greasy, fried and processed venues, which were easy and cheap to prepare couldn't compete. They staged lies and deceit to reduce the old woman's reputation. When this didn't work they expanded their effort to include the local magistrate. This is similar to how chronic inflammation uses vascular inflammatory free radicals to expand an increasingly rogue immune arsenal within interstitial spaces to create an alternative feedback loop system to deceive the capillary cell allies (mesenchymal cells) while isolating the end organ.

The detective's palms were greased by the local eateries compares to how mesenchymal cells are sabotaged (paid off) by alternative feedback loop messages from vagabond immune arsenal.

When the old woman is arrested she is put in jail and her cottage falls into disrepair. This can be compared to how chronic inflammation blocks the capillary cell dance and "imprisons" the capacity of the capillary cell to respond rendering them impotent to an inflammatory assault within interstitial spaces.

As Kate sits in jail and declines, memories of her nutrient rich soups fade and the town folk revert back to the greasy-processed venues of local eateries. As a result, they suffer more pain, fatigue and chronic illnesses.

When Kate is finally released from jail, she reestablishes her previous daily rhythms, which eventually reverses most of her physical and emotional declines she had while being prisoned. Similarly, when vascular inflammatory free radicals are reduced within interstitial spaces, the capillary cells are not pressured to continue trafficking more immune arsenal into the interstitial space and can be released from the confines of the dark and alternative feedback loop systems generated from chronic inflammation. Capillaries can restart their pivot and swing dance, which eventually rebuilds its own feedback loop system to restore interstitial space sanitation. When this occurs, the capillary cell rejuvenates its infrastructure, which is similar to what happens to Kate as she resumes her anti-inflammatory nature walks, foraging and stewing.

As the old woman rejuvenates, the detective switches sides in her favor. Similarly, as the capillary cell resumes its dance and restores its feedback loop system, mesenchymal cells within the interstitial space switch allegiance back to the capillary cell. After the old woman and detective get married, they reopen their patio regularly to locals who return to enjoy the invigorating soups. When the capillary and mesenchymal cells reestablish their feedback loop relationship, they reopen a sanitized interstitial space, which enables the end organ to prosper from increases in blood flow, oxygen and nutrient.

Even a sick old woman can be transformed, if she finds her rejuvenating rhythm. A sick capillary cell can do the same thing if proinflammatory momentum is disrupted by removing vascular inflammatory free radicals, to enable the return of the pivot and swing dance and all the anti-inflammatory momentum that follows.

CHAPTER 4

LIFESTYLE CHOICES: DOWN SHIFTING INFLAMMATORY MOMENTUM BY REDUCING VASCULAR INFLAMMATORY FREE RADICALS

How Lifestyle Choices Work on the Capillary Cell Dance

In any given moment, capillary cell outer membranes are in pro or anti-inflammatory flux. The capillary cell's outer membrane capacity to *flux its outer membrane permeability,* not only helps mastermind its own homeostasis, but paces and stems similar adjustments to the interstitial space, immune arsenal, mesenchymal cells and end organ. With dynamic back and forth fluxing, the rhythm of balancing interstitial space hygiene with optimal end organ function is produced by masterminding an extensive feedback loop system that ties all the moving parts together into a homeostatic rhythm. When this rhythm is optimal, the interstitials space is sanitized and the end organ nurtured. Chronic interstitial space inflammation is subdued as there is no free radical fuel within the interstitial space to do its business.

That being said, chronic inflammation is potentially looming within the interstitial space background waiting to pounce if given enough fuel. This occurs when vascular inflammatory free radicals increase and perpetuate a basement membrane plume of immune arsenal attachments (white blood cells, cytokines, platelets etc.). The perpetuation of immune arsenal expansion into the interstitial space is what strains the capillary cell dance. Without the back and forth outer membrane permeability flux, capillary cell mitochondria get stuck in energy combustion, superoxide free radicals proliferate and capillary cell infrastructure gets blighted. The blocked back and forth pivot and swing dance weakens the capillary cell to where it no longer can implement feedback loop control over the interstitial space or to its allies. The weakened and inept capillary cell feedback loops become the welcome wagon to chronic interstitial space inflammation. As capillary cell feedback loops weaken, chronic inflammatory feedback loops strengthen largely expressed by rogue immune arsenal. There is a new sheriff within the interstitial space, with new feedback loop rules and a different agenda.

Chronic inflammation within interstitial spaces of end organs is *fueled* by vascular inflammatory free radicals and *expanded* by mismatched immune arsenal. The conversion of interstitial space immune arsenal into a rogue force working against capillary cell outer membranes occurs when capillary cells lose their efficiency in sequencing an appropriate immune arsenal. This occurs as their mitochondria and outer membrane receptors diminish from lack of nitric oxide rejuvenation. This proinflammatory momentum chain reacts a chronic inflammatory agenda which stems from establishing its own feedback loop system within the interstitial space utilizing immune arsenal and mesenchymal cell pieces that were formerly allied to the capillary cell. Lifestyle choices has everything to do with how well this malignant interstitial space drama enfolds.

Lifestyle Choices Gone Bad

Most chronic inflammatory transition within interstitial spaces is induced by proinflammatory lifestyle choices. They do so by increasing vascular inflammatory free radicals within interstitial spaces. These free radicals chain react on each other as they partner lifestyle choices which cause more inflammation. It is common for a couch potato to also be sleep deprived and feel more stress. This combination lends itself to snacking, alcohol, sugars, salt and even drugs. Actually any of these can gateway any of the others. Sugar can gateway alcohol, salt, couch potato, sleep deprivation and stress. These behaviors trigger a variety of free radicals that include hormones, toxins, addictions and metabolic exhaust that promulgate free radical fuel into interstitial spaces for chronic inflammation to exploit. The endothelia, which serve as the front line between the blood plasma and to the interstitial spaces of end organs, get caught in the middle of this onslaught and take the brunt of the initial punishment. As basement membranes are impinged and thickened from combinations of free radicals and immune arsenal attachment a permeability trap is set where they can no longer pivot and swing effectively. Mitochondria and outer membrane receptors decline, more mistakes are made involving immune arsenal penetration and before long the interstitial space has become a hostile working environment, replete with its own renegade communication system.

Capillary cell outer membrane permeability in normal homeostasis requires *elimination* of interstitial space inflammatory breach including vascular inflammatory free radicals. Doing so keeps immune arsenal trafficking sequenced and precise as capillary cell outer membrane receptors and mitochondrial volumes rejuvenate from appropriate swinging of mitochondrial combustion to nitric oxide. Trafficking precision enables a kill shot and removal of breach suspects. The execution of the kill shot could involve a variety of trafficked white blood cells, cytokines, immunoglobulins, other inflammatory proteins, complement, platelets or growth factors. *Once removed*, capillary cell outer membranes and mitochondria get a rejuvenating breather by downshifting permeability and swinging combustion ot nitric oxide.

The combustion shift changes capillary cell purpose from sanitizing the interstitial space to nurturing the end organ and rejuvenating its infrastructure. The outer membrane downshift in permeability guarantees that the capillary cell remains effective in its dual purpose. When capillary cell outer membranes flux their permeability, it loops this flux to their mitochondria which chain reacts a host of beneficial outcomes. Not only do capillary cells rejuvenate, but they initiate the tidy withdrawal of immune arsenal from the interstitial space, rejuvenate the mesenchymal cell system, and increase blood flow (oxygen and nutrient) delivery and potential energy combustion to the end organ.

Outcomes of Poor Lifestyle Choices: From Bad to Worse

Once chronic inflammation has formed a matrix and successfully pirated capillary cell outer membranes and gutted their infrastructure chronic inflammation can ride the momentum to control interstitial space signaling. This becomes particularly easy to do when poor lifestyle choices compound, thereby increasing the assault of different free radicals impinging interstitial spaces and basement membranes. Inflammatory momentum progresses when weakened capillary cell feedback loops are replaced enabling the subversion of interstitial space mesenchymal cells to the chronic inflammatory agenda. With capillary cells zombied and interstitial space immune arsenal and mesenchymal cells in tow, chronic inflammation has matured to implement anti-organ disease venues. These venues torture the already disabled end organ to cause further declines and induce waves of pain and fatigue. Scarring, cancer, infections, autoimmune complexes and thrombosis within interstitial spaces occur in waves and in combinations as the true end organ struggles to survive.

At some point, it doesn't matter what poor lifestyle choices have been made. Towards the end of the chronic inflammatory cascade, they all have a similar effect in the interstitial space. Compounding poor lifestyle choices cause these outcomes to occur faster and with more virulence. All of them have in common a blocked capillary cell dance, reduction in mitochondrial volumes and pseudocapillarization of outer membranes. These mechanics don't occur in isolation of one end organ but rather promulgates its effects with interstitial spaces involving all end organs Sleep deprivation, stress, tobacco, sugar, alcohol, drugs, or couch potato status don't just effect the heart, brain and lungs but invade end organ interstitial spaces everywhere. The different diseases that result are co linked by the degradation of the capillary cell and interstitial spaces.

Although pseudocapillarization signals a desperate and gutted capillary cell, it does not necessarily imply a terminal one. Reducing vascular inflammatory free radical burden within interstitial spaces, even in late stages of chronic inflammation, could still produce enough anti-inflammatory momentum to spark a downward shift in capillary cell outer membrane permeability. This would enable a weak but reemerging mitochondrial nitric oxide combustion. If capillary cell mitochondria can find enough impetus to consistently make more nitric oxide, they have impetus to heal.

Making lifestyle changes, to block the chronic inflammatory elephant in the room, starts with knowing the difference between pro and anti-inflammatory behaviors while also acknowledging the gateway risks to these choices. Simple changes like breathing fresh air and drinking clean water are obvious and don't usually require overcoming addictions. Other anti-inflammatory lifestyle gets more difficult as they involve how we move and eat, how we manage pleasure and pain, and how we well we sleep and mitigate stress.

Central to optimal anti-inflammatory adjusting is an awareness of cross reacting addictions to sugar, tobacco, alcohol and drugs and how they gateway an interconnected abuse cycle. Yes, sugar can gateway more sugar, but could also increase risk for alcoholism and even narcotic abuse from sugar induced reductions in pain thresholds. The same interconnected gateways can be said about other addictions. Anti-inflammatory adjustments also involve an understanding about the benefits of regular exercise. Doing it becomes a potent outlier against chronic inflammation. What also be understood is the impact of age itself on proinflammatory momentum and the requirement to become even more stringent in what we choose to expose ourselves to. Everything from a donut to foul air gets magnified with advanced age. With aging, we also tend to sleep lighter and with more interruptions, worry more, move less and are less inclined to engage in healthy eating habits. All of these behavioral trends linked to aging support inflammation.

At the same time, with aging, we must also differentiate benign versus serious symptoms. This means exhibiting proper judgement about what has been nagging and predictable versus what is new and progressive. New symptoms that involve increasing fatigue, pain, shortness of breath, bruising or bleeding, fevers or new lumps should not be ignored. We should submit to at least annual blood work to measure inflammatory markers, blood pressure, pulse, glucose, lipids, thyroid, kidney and liver function, and make sure our vaccines, mammograms and colonoscopies are up to date. Good health requires good judgement, preparation, paying attention to changes in our bodies, and most important, more intentional anti-inflammatory behaviors. In addition to selective medicinals, adding in supplements, including antioxidants and vitamin D, among others, will likely be required. It must also be understood that there are no short cuts when it comes to food quality and preparation.

The consciousness of lifestyle choices should be based on the awareness that chronic inflammatory momentum increases with age and must be addressed with an equal assault against it. Every lifestyle decision should be based on a conscious risk-benefit attempt to block chronic inflammation. For more details about the dos and do nots of lifestyle choices, extensive discussions can be found in my two previous books, *Hazing Aging* (I- Universe 2015) and *Rejuvenation!* (I-Universe 2017).

CHAPTER 5

THE PLANTING AND GROWTH OF CHRONIC INFLAMMATION

The birthing of chronic interstitial space inflammation begins with persistent vascular inflammatory free radical infiltration as a result of poor lifestyle choices and further accentuated by inherited or malfunctioned genes. The *Trafficking* glossary provides two different graphs highlighting the relationship of behavioral choices, age and the subsequent increases in hemoglobin A1C and advanced glycation end products. In truth any vascular inflammatory free radical could be plugged into this curve and it would look the same. The curve becomes in graph 2 shifts to the left as additional vascular free radicals are added to the mix, meaning that disease venues and likely mortality emerge much sooner in life. Implied in free radical emergence within interstitial spaces, are the repeated patterns of a blocked capillary cell dance, the eventual dispersal of a random and rogue immune arsenal, and the unleashing of a dark and alternative feedback loop cascade. As this occurs, the capillary cell capitulates and chronic inflammation seizes control of the interstitial space. Graph 3 in the glossary demonstrates the different stages of chronic inflammation and the eventual deployment of disease venues.

How Vascular Free Radicals Cause Importation of Rebel Immune Arsenal

Just as anti-inflammatory behaviors tend to feed off of each other to improve interstitial space sanitation and promote wellness, the reverse also occurs. Different vascular inflammatory free radicals can play off of each other through addictions, stress, sleep deprivation, and couch potato status to cause a gathering of proinflammatory interstitial space momentum. As they aggregate a well- diversified portfolio of free radicals, they attach to basement membranes, *induce* permeability adjustments on capillary cell outer membranes, to commandeer immune arsenal entry into the interstitial space towards their attachment. Unfortunately, their persistence derails the capillary cell's capacity to continue sending a sequenced immune arsenal towards them. As mitochondria overheat, increase superoxide exhaust, and decapitate their DNA, they increasingly commit suicide and their volumes within the cell diminish. This cascades to include an outer membrane collapse, as receptors, voltage gradients and pores all diminish in unison. Before you know it the capillary cell can no longer choreograph. Trafficking of immune arsenal becomes random which places the interstitial space up for grabs as to who or what controls white blood cell release of cytokines and other inflammatory mediators. None of this plays out well for the interstitial space or end organ.

As capillary cell feedback loops disintegrate the slack is picked up by the evolving chronic inflammatory matrix as it utilizes the signaling glitches created by the preexisting and random interstitial space immune arsenal to its advantage. As rebel cytokine signaling increases, the rogue feedback loop momentum is picked up by interstitial space mesenchymal cells as they become the last group of cells within the interstitial space to switch allegiance from the dysfunctional capillary cell network towards the coalesced inflammatory matrix. Together with converted mesenchymal cells, they foray an interstitial space alliance of proinflammatory momentum enabling chronic inflammation to further expand influence to include disease venues.

The Attack and Stacking Effect

It could be hypothesized said that each *unmitigated* vascular inflammatory free radical could cost 5 years of lost life span. *Multiple or stacked* unmitigated vascular inflammatory free radicals could reduce lifespan by 20 or more years. As an example, a current smoker and alcoholic, who also happens to be a diabetic with elevated blood plasma LDL cholesterol, could expect life expectancy to be cut short by as many as 30 years! The shortened lifespan is also accompanied by chronic pain, fatigue, numerous medications, tests and surgeries, and serious physical limitations prior to death. The physical breakdown is often accompanied by dementia and a host of different specialists and medicines required to treat pain, fatigue and medical conditions. The medical industrial complex is kept busy by these lost souls who are constantly utilizing services from new and evolving problems. Their premature demise is usually accompanied by dependency, diapers and dementia.

Many of the stacked interconnected proinflammatory behaviors are *addiction based*, meaning they seamlessly gateway each other. Nicotine addiction from smoking cigarettes may gateway connections to alcohol, sugar or salt. All of these lead to chronic pain which then introduces opioid narcotics to the mix. Together they numb the brain into thinking all is ok while they do their deception within interstitial spaces. At some point, we no longer have the capacity to mount enough mental fortitude to fight them off and they just take over. They become the perfect mechanism for chronic inflammation to exert interstitial space control.

First and Second Line Inflammatory Mediators: Birds of a Feather?

To clarify, vascular inflammatory free radicals have been discussed and defined in detail in my book *Rejuvenation!* They are also known as *first-line vascular inflammatory mediator-risks* or as *vascular free radical interstitial space and basement membrane seeds*. They initiate the inflammatory process by penetrating through endothelia outer membranes to enter the interstitial spaces of end organs, and then do their inflammatory business by attaching to basement membranes or other cell surfaces within the space. Once attached to a membrane they trigger an inflammatory expansion by immune arsenal for the purpose of their expulsion from the membrane. This trafficked expansion of immune arsenal into the interstitial space is known as the *second line of vascular inflammatory mediators.* This diverse group of inflammatory mediators can arrive at the inflammatory staging area from blood plasma or lymph vessels and participate in removal of the offending particle, molecule, toxin or other free radical. Their success triggers the endothelia outer membranes to decrease permeability and swing combustion to nitric oxide, thereby allowing capillary and endothelial cells the opportunity to stay effective in sanitizing the interstitial spaces.

Depending on what vascular inflammatory free radical seeds the interstitial space, will determine what kind of immune arsenal attack is sequenced by the endothelia. By changing up their outer membrane receptors, pores, and voltage gradients, endothelia can usher into the interstitial space different blends of anti-inflammatory proteins, cytokines, white blood cells, clotting factors and platelets with the sole purpose of eliminating the offending inflammatory breach. If for any reason the removal process backfires, chronic inflammation gains an opening as the endothelia must extend permeability and energy combusting efforts to further attempt inflammatory breach removal. This becomes the first crack in endothelial and capillary cell armor.

The backfire becomes much more likely when vascular inflammatory free radical seeds stack within interstitial spaces, as evidenced by *addictive* proinflammatory lifestyles and choices. When vascular inflammatory free radical seeds, are both well- diversified and abundant within interstitial spaces, the risks for chronic inflammation will increase substantially. As previously discussed, addictions to sugar, alcohol, tobacco, and drugs can gateway each other and are perfect interludes to this kind of well diversified proinflammatory assault on interstitial spaces. As this occurs, cracks in endothelial and capillary infrastructure occur as their mitochondria get stuck in energy combustion and they begin producing too much superoxide exhaust, which cannot be effectively neutralized. The proinflammatory chain reactions eventually claim capillary cell outer membrane receptors and infrastructure thereby nullifying immune arsenal sequencing in favor of random and error prone dispersal into interstitial spaces.

How Chronic Inflammation Eviscerates the Capillary Cell

The chronic inflammatory interstitial space free fall is ushered in by the blocked capillary cell pivot-pendulum swing dance. Over time the blocked dance eviscerates the capillary cell from the inside out rendering it incapable of any meaningful sequencing of immune arsenal or effective responses to end organ energy requirements. The interstitial space becomes a hostile place where mesenchymal cells must cease, desist and convert to a different and darker array of feedback loop signals. Eventually chronic inflammation creates enough feedback loops momentum to establish disease venues, which define the anti-organ.

Every cell, enzyme, clotting factor and protein that the endothelia had at its sequencing disposal and controlled by powerful feedback loop relationships between interstitial space white blood, mesenchymal and end organ cells becomes subverted and deceptively used for alternative purposes by chronic inflammation. This means the downstream endothelia and upstream capillary cells have been subjugated by the breakdown of their infrastructure and the subsequent diversion of their signaling influences to an alternative-and contrary signaling system devised by chronic inflammation. As chronic inflammation subverts and twists feedback loop messages within the interstitial spaces utilizing rogue immune arsenal, the momentum of random trafficking through the capillary cell becomes easier thereby enabling disease venues to nurture. As this occurs, the true end organ becomes increasingly dysfunctional as disease venues, aging, pain and fatigue escalate. Not only does cancer, infections and thrombosis proliferate but so do disease outcomes that involve dementia, blindness, hearing loss, heart, lung and kidney failure, fatty liver, disabling arthritis, and increasing malabsorption as all end organs take proinflammatory hits from the diffuse assault on interstitial spaces involving the entire vascular tree.

Vascular Free Radicals Rarely show their Cards Early

Why are vascular inflammatory free radicals so sinister? The short answer is because they can be *prevalent, addictive, and work in combinations* to do much of their early damage to interstitial spaces and basement membranes in *stealth mode*. Extensive interstitial space damage and capillary-endothelial cell damage can occur before any signs or symptoms emerge. This makes vascular inflammatory free radical seeds dangerous as early their progression is not often signaled.

Most of the time, free radical seeds only "show themselves" after the afflicted end organ(s) have well established disease venues that are producing disabling symptoms.

Vascular inflammatory free radicals are ubiquitous and be a toxic gas, particle, toxin, or a metabolic byproduct of end organ combustion. It can take on many shapes, sizes and forms. It can come from the air we breathe, water we drink, food we eat, stress we endure or sleep we don't get. In some cases, free radicals are excessively produced by our own end organs based on aberrant genetics. Examples include advanced glycation end products, C reactive protein (or highly sensitive C reactive protein), small particle LDL cholesterol, lipoprotein (a), apolipoprotein B, and homocysteine among several others. All of these can produce proinflammatory cascades in stealth mode for year within interstitial spaces before symptoms emerge.

The Addiction "Gateway" Effect

To understand the addiction –free radical seeding process, let's choose smoking a cigarette and the nicotine addiction that it causes. Dragging on a cigarette, cigar or pipe, in addition to inhaling nicotine, also unleashes at least 16 additional free radicals into our lungs and throat from the inhaled smoke. Many of these inhaled toxins are capable of easy migration through mucus membranes or lung alveolar cells into interstitial spaces. Once there, they can migrate into capillaries and then into the blood stream where they get disseminated throughout the body. As they move in and out of cells they cause a disruptive path that begins with their initial contact with the lung and capillary cell outer membranes. They can further disrupt cell infrastructure by attaching to different membrane surfaces of organelles or disrupting mitochondrial combustion. Once they enter the blood stream, they can affect the entire vascular tree, their interstitial spaces and multiple end organs. Since nicotine is highly addictive and creates both pleasure craving and a painful withdrawal, it is a foregone conclusion that smoking more cigarettes will occur to perpetuate pleasure and prevent withdrawal. These addiction characteristics can also occur from sugar, opioids, sleeping pills, anti-anxiety medicines, alcohol and stimulants. When used in sequence or together, there proinflammatory effects escalate an even stronger *pleasure-withdrawal* cascade, but now they can involve several different chemicals or toxins. And each can gateway another.

As addictions progress, the user becomes oblivious to what is occurring as the brain shuts down to normal logic in favor of finding more pleasure or limiting withdrawal. This is when the user has typically coupled several addictions and has started the process of losing friends, spouses, and jobs. Multiple different end organ disease venues pop-up as endothelial and capillary cell basement membranes throughout the arterial tree thicken and they stop dancing. With different disease venues comes chronic pain, fatigue and accelerated aging as teeth fall out, muscles atrophy, joints stiffen, breathlessness increases and the brain fries.

Addictions cause *tolerance* meaning you have to use more to get the same or desired effect. All this does is escalate chronic inflammation, and further increase the risk for serious withdrawal symptoms, which further imprisons the user. So, one of everything becomes two and then three cigarettes, donuts, beers, bags of potato chips, opioids, amphetamines or sleeping pills. As we eat, drink, snort, inject, pop or smoke, we need even more to get less benefit. This equation of spiraling dependency sets in motion loss of jobs, relationships, finances and personal hygiene. The street becomes home with a premature morgue visit becoming the final destination.

The Sugar Conundrum

The sugar addiction problem is complex because of how many simple sugars spike our foods and drinks. A common misconception is that all sugar is sweet. In reality most simple sugars are not sweet. The sugar problem has escalated through food processing and deceptive labeling practices. *Any* simple sugar can increase sugar addiction and can serve as a gateway to other addictions. Sugar is found in table sugar (sucrose) and fructose (or fructose corn syrup) and is commonly added to candy, juices, coffee creamers, colas, cereals, yogurts, accoutrements (ketchup) or canned fruits. Simple sugars, such as lactose, are not sweet can be found in dairy products. Highly processed bread, pasta and corn products have high quantities of sugar but don't taste sweet. Alcoholic beverages of all kinds are very high in sugar, with beer demonstrating the most sugar per serving.

Sugar labeling is often deceptive as it may only count sucrose or table sugar as sugar grams. This means that most other sugars are either not counted or labelled as "other" when counting carbohydrate grams per serving. When looking at package labelling, if total carbohydrates are X, and the total fiber and sugar grams don't add up to X, make the assumption that the discrepancy is from hidden sugars that were not counted.

All sugars, whether sweet or not, *cross effect* meaning as a class they don't block *satiety* or a feeling of being full or calorie satisfied. This enables sugar ingestion to increase risk for overeating or even binge eating. In western culture this is why eating a sugary dessert coupled with a sweet liquor at the end of a meal is easily consumed. In spite of being satisfied and certainly not hungry there is always "room" for dessert or an after dinner drink or both.

Simple sugars are commonplace, and associated with very high advanced glycemic indexes in highly processed snack foods, cereals, breads, rice, and pastas. Anything processed, packaged, and frequently salted from a chip to a bagel contains abundant highly processed white flour. In this manner, even without being sweet, eating a bagel, cold cereal, or snacking on a chip or cracker is *feeding* sugar addiction, will contribute to weight gain and subliminally increase desire for more sugar. .

The point being that snacking on a cracker or a chip may seem harmless but can subliminally gateway sugar addiction to binging or overeating. This can mean that a glass of wine or a beer could subliminally increase cravings for chips, crackers, cheese, a bagel or visa- versa. Even worse, the subliminal cravings could persist for hours, maybe days. Because of this convergence, sugars not only trigger more sugar but could gateway other addictions by multiplying the comfort-pleasure withdrawal equation from caffeine, nicotine, opioids, or amphetamines. Over the last 50 years, upwards of 75% of supermarket inventory could be sugar based. It is not any wonder that in this 50 year stretch one in 3 Americans adults have become either obese or morbidly obese from the effects of sugar addiction. And sugar substitutes are no better as they continue to feed the subliminal desires for more sugar.

The "Aging Effect" of Addiction's Triple Double

Inflammatory expansion into end organ interstitial spaces caused from addictive habits triples from age 25 to 65. One cigarette, donut, beer or strip of bacon at age 65 is the equivalent of *3 of the same at age 25*. This is due to age related lingering of free radicals released into interstitial spaces. Eating one donut may spike blood sugars for 3-4 hours in a 65-year-old but maybe for 60 minutes in a fit 25-year-old. The persistent spike in blood sugars triggers chain reactions of proinflammatory effects that can last until blood sugars finally decrease in the blood. The same is true with inhaling the hydrocarbons from a cigarette or metabolizing alcohol. With aging, we become less efficient in elimination of these toxins form our blood stream, which gives them longer periods of time to act as free radicals, enter interstitial spaces, and induce hate crimes in the interstitial space. Hence these habits, particularly when age adjusted, *accelerate* chronic inflammation and disease venues within interstitial spaces. Smoking even 5 cigarettes a day at age 65 will dramatically increase risk for COPD as well as many different cancers compared to smoking at 25.

The proinflammatory effects of nicotine, opioids, amphetamines, sugar, caffeine, trans-fat and salt increase dramatically with aging and will shorten life span by years to decades. This risk accelerates further when these addictions couple.

As addictions blend and gateway others, multiple end organ disease venues mount, from infections, cancer and scarring to thrombosis and autoimmune complex disease. All too often disease treatment facilitates other diseases or treatment complications thereby compounding medical dilemmas, increasing expense and forcing the pinball effect, of bouncing form one doctor, procedure and treatment to another, in an endless transition within the medical industrial complex. Meanwhile as treatments fatigue and pain escalate, a computer is required to keep track of medications, diseases, tests, procedures and appointments. In many cases, the right hand does not know what the left hand is doing, as doctors scurry to document their electronic medical records manifesto without bothering to call or communicate with other doctors about treatment plans.

We need to have a much better awareness of the big picture when it comes to proliferating care in the disease treatment model. Again, I harken back to a better understanding of how chronic inflammation transitions and how this should be our method of choice in preventing these terrible disease outcomes (see appendix graph 3).

The Buddying Up of Aging, Chronic Inflammation and Capillary Cell Mitochondrial Energy Combustion

Why does aging make chronic inflammation more likely? The aging effect against inflammation is like playing a game of basketball with only one hand. In gets twice as hard to defend, let alone dribble or shoot. With regards to endothelia, because of age related accumulation of DNA damage, there are built in inefficiencies within the cell's infrastructure, outer membranes and mitochondria. Ineffective genetic coding for protein synthesis, whether for replacement or repair, have silenced certain outer membrane receptor proteins, or those involved in mitochondria combustion or other organelles. When proteins no longer function, regardless of where, these structure within or outside of the cell are less effective in what they do, meaning they perform less efficiently. For any given inflammatory breach, aging makes outer membrane receptors and mitochondrial energy combustion *less responsive* thereby increasing risk for ineffective clearing and subsequent chronic inflammation.

DNA coding errors increase mistakes in protein synthesis, which marginalizes the capillary cell's capacity to receive and respond to signals involving inflammatory breach, mesenchymal or end organ cells. It also inherently weakens its feedback loop system between its interstitial space partners, thereby predisposing to its pirating by chronic inflammation.

So aging, by biasing inhibition of capillary cell repair and replacement can stem a similar debacle with adjacent mesenchymal and somatic cells. Given this context, aging blends nicely with vascular inflammatory free radical fuel to induces a rapid spirals of capillary and end organ cellular decline. The coupling of increasing capillary cell incompetence with abundant free radical fuel becomes a perfect interstitial space breeding ground for chronic inflammation. The antidote for this ugly convergence is an even more stringent limit placed on free radical exposures. With aging, there is no such thing as a little bit of this or that. This is true when choices are linked to sugar, tobacco, animal fats or being a couch potato.

Stem cell transplants into endothelial, capillary and end organs may offer some help in reversing age related DNA damage to lessen silenced protein production. Unless they are accompanied by rigorous lifestyle adjustments, the other side of the equation involving capillary cell nitric oxide driven rejuvenation, will not occur and no amount of stem cell intervention will have long term benefit.

With a clear understanding of how chronic inflammation nests within interstitial spaces, it would seem an obvious fit for older people to go all in, but sadly in western cultures the opposite occurs. We appear to gladly give in to bulging waistlines, as we take an extra piece of cake and sip on a diet coke. These combinations tsunami a vascular inflammatory free radical surges thereby pushing elevations in blood pressures and sugars and all the free radical fall-out that follows. The proinflammatory dominos fall in rapid succession as increasing pain, fatigue and incipient dementia fast track increased confusion and dependency. Instead of facing free radical challenges for what they are, we gladly give into them. As we walk into the valley of the shadow of death, the chronic inflammatory anti-organ has prepared a devastating last chapter for us that usually involves a tortured existence of dependency, dementia and diapers coupled with chronic pain and fatigue. We collaborate on an end game we never wanted or intended.

What Confers a Vascular Inflammatory Free Radical?

Table one below highlights different vascular inflammatory free radicals and basic proinflammatory mechanics. Some of these highlights involve disease venues with several vascular inflammatory free radicals, while others, like sleep deprivation or stress, produce free radicals indirectly through the release of stress hormones. Regardless of having a direct or indirect effect on free radical expansion within interstitial spaces, the collection below samples the connections of lifestyle to free radical delivery.

Table One

The First Wave of Inflammatory Assault: A Cause-Effect List of Vascular Inflammatory Free Radicals

1. Diabetes Mellitus - A disease manifestation of too much glucose (pyruvate), fatty acid energy substrate that increases free radical LDL cholesterol, and AGE-free radicals, (advanced glycation end products) to attach and inflame outer membranes. Leads to chronic interstitial space inflammation to involve all end organs.

2. LDL Cholesterol - Sticky free radical (ox-small particle LDL)-adheres to membrane surfaces to plume chronic inflammation.

3. Tobacco - Carbon monoxide gas plus 16 or more toxins from inhaled smoke disrupt endothelial and capillary cell membrane surfaces to spiral interstitial space inflammation. Linked to nicotine addiction and disease venues involving multiple end organs.

4. Trans- fats - Incorporate, disable and plume endothelial and capillary cell outer membranes to induce chronic inflammation.

5. Hypertension - A disease venue linked to elevated blood sugars, LDL cholesterol, AGEs, diabetes, tobacco use, and inactivity. Damages endothelia by increasing shear stress to effect multiple end organs.

6. Triglycerides - Increases fatty acid energy substrate, and endothelial and capillary cell outer membrane inflammation. Increased blood levels, causes and effects are similar to diabetes.

7. Lipoprotein (a) - Sticky non HDL cholesterol substance-adheres to and inflames endothelial and capillary cell outer membrane surfaces. Often genetically increased, linked to hypoxic ischemic events (heart attacks, strokes, vascular dementia and aortic valve stenosis).

8. Homocysteine - Sticky molecule that adheres to membrane surfaces to cause inflammation. Increased blood levels with age. Linked to thrombosis, strokes and vascular dementia.

9. Pro-Coagulants - Increase clotting and platelet aggregation through a variety of mechanisms. Linked to inheritance and disease venues that include cancer, autoimmune and infectious diseases. risk for hypoxic-ischemic events such as heart attacks, deep vein leg clots, lung clots (pulmonary emboli) and strokes.

10. Drugs — Expanding list of prescribed and street drugs, inflame capillary cell outer membranes, and increase free radicals. Examples include prolonged use of steroids, methamphetamines for ADHD and proton pump acid blockers for GERD.

11. Alcohol — Alcohol is metabolized similarly to sugar, and plumes endothelial outer membrane inflammation with similar causes and effects. In excess it marginalizes interstitial spaces, toxifies multiple end organs to cause several disease venues.

12. Stress — Increases stress hormones linked to cascading endothelial outer membrane inflammation through multiple pathways to increase risk for disease venues including thrombosis, infectious diseases and cancer.

13. Sleep Disturbances — Similar to stress, causes increase in stress hormones.

14. Social isolation — Mimics the effects of stress, often by perpetuating addictions and other aberrant behaviors.

15. Immobility — Plumes endothelial outer membrane inflammation through several proinflammatory pathways, increasing risks for obesity, sarcopenia and adult diabetes.

16. Addictions — to drugs, tobacco, alcohol, produce unwanted toxicity to endothelial cell outer membranes, interstitial spaces and end organs leading to multiple disease venues.

18. Toxins/particulates — Can act as free radicals to plume endothelial outer membranes inflammation or have a direct effect on infrastructure. The list of toxins is expanding and includes among others arsenic, mercury, lead, aluminum, asbestosis, insecticides, pesticides, toxic gases as well as multiple other chemicals. Chronic exposures produce multiple disease venues including end organ scarring, cancers, infections and thrombosis.

Vascular inflammatory free radicals like to buddy up to double down interstitial space impingement, hence their interconnectedness. Whether from addictions, or for other reasons involving laziness, comfort or pleasure, poor lifestyle choices breed more of the same to eventually concoct an interstitial space stew that becomes the highway to hell.

The Logistics of Pseudocapillarization

Pseudocapillarization occurs when the capillary cell's infrastructure can no longer support outer membrane function. Mitochondrial volumes shrink and nuclear DNA coding mistakes increase to a point, where even if protein synthesis does occur, the manufactured proteins are either silent or function in competently. To outer membranes of endothelia, it means the drying up of infrastructure, receptors, pores, voltage gradients and capacity to elicit vesicles and transport channels. In short, the capacity to stage an immune arsenal response to inflammatory to diminished to the extent that their receptors, pore density and energy support will allow. Inevitably this translates into improper entrance of the wrong immune arsenal into the interstitial space staging area of inflammatory breach. The mistakes self-perpetuate to where enough contrary proinflammmatory momentum builds within the interstitial space to challenge the feedback loops of the ailing capillary cell. As this occurs pseudocapillarization has thickened the basement membrane from the effects of chronic inflammation, thinned the glycocalyx, and reduced the continuous outer membrane to a shell of what it once was. Thus pseudocapillariation becomes an expected outcome to chronic inflammation.

This threshold for accelerated chronic inflammatory momentum becomes dependent on the degree of pseudocapillarization that has occurred, the vascular inflammatory free radical fuel, and the disease venues that have been enabled. As all of these thresholds increase, proinflammatory momentum accelerates. Of the three, the only way to incur a reversal is to shut down the fuel source.

Pseudocapillarization of capillary cell outer membranes becomes an urgent red flag signaling a dying endothelial -capillary cell and implying chronic inflammatory feedback loop control of the interstitial space. Mitochondrial volumes have shrunk, nitric oxide combustion only trickles at best, and nuclear DNA has likely become severely compromised. It becomes the white flag to surrendering their feedback loops relationships to their interstitial space partners, including the end organ.

Pseudocapillarization of capillary cell outer membranes becomes the kill shot of the chronic inflammatory matrix. Once it takes down the capacity for capillary cells to sequence immune arsenal, the coast becomes clear for chronic inflammation to assemble a rebel group of immune white blood cells, platelets and immunoglobulins. As this rebel group increases in stature it becomes its own interstitial space force to be reckoned with. As capillary cell feedback loops surrender, chronic inflammation matures and refines its intent by unleashing disease venues. This becomes the calling card for progressive end organ failure as aging, fatigue and pain begin in earnest.

Epigenetics

Epigenetics, or how we choose to live our life, can become an antidote or poison to our genetics. If choices are beneficial to our capillaries, we frame wellness and lessen the impact of our genetic vulnerabilities. Poor life style choices will do the opposite. The implication is that the way we choose to live could trump a disparaged genetic profile or keep weaker genes in hiding for much longer periods of time. This means that lifestyle could override such common inherited diseases as diabetes, heart disease, cancer, arthritis or dementia, to name a few.

The revelation of how epigenetics can effect aging is taking on increasing interest asitI relates to mitigating chronic inflammation. A lifestyle overhaul coupled with timely interventions of supplements and medicinals could block or slow down disease venue manifestations for decades. In other words, implementing beneficial epigenetics could influence disease outcomes more than genetic predisposition. If we eat right, exercise, sleep well, mitigate stress and practice good preventative health care, we stand a good chance of dodging, at least for much longer periods, what our parents or grandparents died from.

This is particularly true when it comes to addictions. Lifestyle choices that block *gateway exposures* to sugar, drugs, tobacco and alcohol could mastermind or postpone an entirely different set of outcomes that occurred through generations of the family tree. Making these lifestyle choices *earlier,* greatly improves chances of blocking an inherited foil.

This theory presupposes that lifestyle interventions work by dramatically reducing vascular inflammatory free radical fuel, thereby limiting the risk of a flip to an adverse genetic on switch. Keeping interstitial spaces sanitized, while not guaranteeing a genetic mishap, gives the capillary cell and infrastructure a leg up in mitigating a genetic vulnerability.

If an adverse genetic profile within a family tree shows an obvious bias to certain diseases, mitigating the free radical fuel early in the next generation should be a priority. Attacking the free radical inflammatory seeds contributing to premature diseases should be an early preventative focus. If there are generations of obese diabetics within a family tree that are dying of stroke and heart attack, changing outcomes in offspring should occur early in life and should include education about diet, exercise and sleep. Otherwise genetics wins. The same can be said about lipid disorders, addictions cancer or autoimmune disease. It makes no sense to pretend that genetic destinies don't matter.

Reactive Oxygen Species and Nuclear DNA Fall-Out

When chronic inflammation establishes an interstitial space foothold, capillary cell mitochondrial combustion gets stuck in energy which causes a reciprocal end organ mitochondrial combustion being stuck in in nitric oxide. Both energy and nitric oxide combustion, when stuck, causes accumulation of toxic free radical exhaust, known as *reactive oxygen species or ROS*. As it gets produced, it burns through available anti-oxidants and begins to accumulate within cells. In the capillary cell the ROS is superoxide, whereas in end organ cells the ROS is biased towards hydroxynitriles, which are cousins to cyanide. These different ROS exhaust bi-products can do harm to membrane surfaces but also have a significant impact on nuclear and mitochondrial DNA. With chronic inflammation, the capillary cell nuclear DNA telomere cap dissipates, as telomerase, the enzyme that reproduces the cap, goes on hiatus. As the telomere cap shortens, more chromosomal DNA gets exposed to free radical cross-linkage, including superoxide. The subsequent superoxide induced cross linkage damages nuclear DNA and causes coding mistakes. These mistakes get reflected when the capillary cell attempts to manufacture proteins for repair and replacement.

The coding mistakes and the incompetent proteins that result form the basis for mitochondrial departure and reduced outer membrane receptors. The combination is a boon to chronic inflammation as it has much more wiggle room to push its agenda within the interstitial space. As nuclear DNA fails, the fall-out magnifies the ineptness of capillary cell outer membrane trafficking of immune arsenal, thereby accelerating an increasingly dark and hostile interstitial space environment.

Can DNA self-repair? The answer means everything in ultimately reversing the aging vortex. Regardless of what stem cells may offer in addressing this question, without a deep clean of interstitial space vascular inflammatory free radicals, any heroic attempts to replace a battered DNA with a newer variety will be just a band aide. For any treatment on DNA to be successful, the interstitial space should be sanitized first to legitimize the capacity of the capillary cell to protect its DNA through nitric oxide driven telomerase activity.

Scarring: The Signature of the Anti-Organ

Interstitial space–end organ scarring is the signature interstitial space sign that chronic inflammation is in control of the interstitial space. The implication is that chronic inflammation has garnered enough interstitial space feedback loop momentum to dupe mesenchymal cells into secreting fibrous scar tissue or amyloid, which serves as a barrier between already dysfunctional capillary and atrophying end organ cells. Precipitation of fibrous scar tissue implies that mesenchymal cells no longer are responding to capillary cell feedback loops, but instead are now going to the beat of a different feedback loop drummer. The basis for the mesenchymal cell split is how deficient capillary cells have become is their feedback loop signaling coupled with the increasing power of an alternative signaling system generated by the chronic inflammatory matrix and rebel immune arsenal. In this setting the capillary cell dance has long been blocked or has become irrelevant to the interstitial space and has been replaced by anew signaling network that is dictating what mesenchymal cells should do.

The scar barrier not only further suffocates the end organ from oxygen and nutrient, but also fosters an interstitial space environment conducive to other disease venues. With the induction of scar tissue the anti-organ can use its crevices and crypts to hide viruses, bacteria, rogue autoimmune complexes, and even cancer cells, which blend into with the scar network as they grow and multiply undetected. It is not uncommon for scarred interstitial spaces to harbor increased risk for serious infections, autoimmune disease, cancers and even thrombotic events. In this manner, scarring supports other disease venues which in turn support more scarring. They are all fueled by vascular inflammatory free radicals.

Can scarring be reversed? It may depend on the degree of collateral damage that scarring has caused within the interstitial space. For any chance of reversal, vascular free radicals must be reduced in order the capillary cells to find their dance footing. If the capillary cell dance is remastered, inflammatory momentum can shift and then the possibility of scar reversal is possible. This is where lifestyle, stem cells and capillary-endothelial cell DNA resurgence must comingle in future studies. The affected end organ will be grateful.

Feedback Loop Cross-Talk Momentum: Who's in Control?

When the interstitial space is in harmony, feedback loops cross talk is occurring vigorously and is led by capillary cell pivot and swing dance involving its outer membranes and mitochondria. Its feedback loop partners include immune arsenal, downstream endothelial and end organs, their adjacent capillary cell colleagues, and their interstitial space allies, the mesenchymal and end organ cells. The outcome is a seamless management of interstitial space sanitation, counterbalanced by optimizing end organ function, all while pacing the regeneration of worn out infrastructure. Immune arsenal is strategically looped into an interstitial space strategy of selective choreography based on need and are then removed. In contrast as immune arsenal comes and goes from the interstitial space, the capillary cell is simultaneously pacing renewal of infrastructure as well as providing the end organ with more oxygen and nutrient for its mitochondrial combustion. The powerful reach of capillary cell feedback loop signaling extends to affect all of its allies in the stemming and pacing of renewal and improved function. These signaling feedback loops are called *cross talk*, are often driven by the release of different cytokines, and form the basis of how capillary cells communicate with their allied partners.

Effective cross talk requires capillary cell outer membrane flux. Without balanced fluxing, feedback loops signals can chain react a colossal breakdown of interstitial space homeostasis. The breakdown keys the script of chronic inflammation.

Mesenchymal Cells-The Last Bastion of Interstitial Space Defense

Mesenchymal cells are critical capillary cell partners in sanitizing the interstitial space. They are found in all end organ interstitial spaces and accessorize the capacity of capillary cells to defend the interstitial space from different invaders ranging from vascular free radicals to cancer cells and infectious agents. Collectively, mesenchymal cells diversity into different roles depending of prevailing interstitial space circumstances. They can act as *scouts* to collect intelligence about what had invaded the interstitial space. Others can execute a *direct attack* on a foreign invader of inflammatory free radicals, while still others can engulf a *tagged* vascular free radical, cancer cell or infectious agent and degrade them into smaller pieces. In other arrangements mesenchymal cells can assist in tagging foreign invaders thereby setting up kill shots by other white blood cells such as lymphocytes or monocytes. When in the hands of chronic inflammation, mesenchymal cells can do all of this same work against rather than for the capillary cell and its end organ partner. In addition, it will produce and secrete generous amounts of fibrous scar tissue or amyloid into the interstitial space to further alienate the disabled capillary cell from its atrophied end organ partner. Mesenchymal cells will respond regardless of where the cross talk originates from.

Mesenchymal cells have different names based on where they are found and what they do within interstitial spaces. Examples include *macrophages, fibrocytes, stellate cells, pericytes, structural connective tissue cells, glial cells (also known as astrocytes among others in the brain) or Kupffer cells (liver)*. Through their different functions, they act as both a *buffer* and *special assistant* to the capillary cell's capacity to provide seamless immune resources to the interstitial space.

When chronic inflammation occurs within the interstitial space, and the capillary cell dance breaks down to where they lose their feedback loop signaling mojo, their crosstalk with all cells including mesenchymal cells becomes unhinged. As expected this creates a usurping of a clearly defined mesenchymal cell purpose and an opportunity for an alternative crosstalk signaling system to be invoked. This becomes *a fait accompli*, as rebel uncommitted immune arsenal infiltrate and disrupt the interstitial space feedback loop network.

As a result of these immune arsenal rebels, mesenchymal cells will convert to the most dominant feedback loop signaling apparatus, which in chronic inflammation favors those cytokine signals released from wayward white blood cells and platelets within the interstitial space. In this manner abundant vascular inflammatory free radical fuel blocks the capillary cell dance, disables the capillary cell and invites a rogue immune arsenal into the interstitial space, which then seizes control of the feedback loop communication system. The threshold for choreographed immune displays within the interstitial space precipitously declines as cross talk radicalizes the space into a more chaotic mosaic. With enough cross talk momentum, mesenchymal cells from friend to foe. Disease venues are in the rear view mirror.

The End Organ No-Man's Land

As chronic inflammation grips the interstitial space, the disease venues it eventually creates strangle the capillary-end organ cell relationship. As rogue feedback loop crosstalk enables disease venues, end organ viability is marginalized. This is brought about from oxygen and nutrient supplies being diverted from the end organ to the burgeoning array of different disease venues. The zombied capillary cell can have minimal impact on this process as long as its dance is blocked by vascular inflammatory free radical fuel that is pummeling the interstitial space and endothelial basement membranes. As the end organ asphyxiates waves of fatigue and pain dominate the clinical landscape. This complete and utter destitution of the interstitial space to an environment completely hostile to the end organ defines the *end organ's no man's land*. All momentum within the interstitial space has shifted to favor chronic inflammation.

The march of chronic inflammatory control of the interstitial space occurs at some level in all end organs interstitial spaces simultaneously. This means, that while one end organ may be grabbing clinical headlines by critically falling below a minimal threshold of function, all end organs are likely being impinged at some level by the same chronic inflammatory processes. Preventing any end organ's, *no man's land* requires an abrupt termination of the free radical fuel that has birthed the chronic inflammatory progression. Nipping vascular inflammatory free radicals early rather than late in the chronic inflammatory process becomes key to preventing the dark reshaping of the interstitial space.

An Ounce of Prevention is Equals to....

Reversing chronic inflammatory momentum within interstitial spaces of end organs gets more difficult as it takes over more control of the crosstalk signals. At any given moment there is a pitch battle of forces within the interstitial space that are working for or against the capillary cell and its allied partners. Unfortunately, father time and the persistent pummeling of the interstitial space by vascular inflammatory free radicals favors the breakdown of the capillary cell dance. To the extent that capillary cells break down and lose feedback loop control of the interstitial space, is to the extent that the space and end organ capitulates to chronic inflammation. As disease venues proliferate, the capacity for capillary and endothelial cell recovery becomes less likely. This occurs for many different reason but usually comes down to too much capillary cell DNA damage which permanently impairs coding and silences protein synthesis for replacement of outer membrane receptors and mitochondrial volumes. Without the regeneration of these two critical pieces, the capillary will not recover enough mojo to stem proinflammatory momentum. Implied in this discussion is that with aging because of already accumulated DNA damage and silenced protein synthesis, there is no lifestyle room for making bad choices without paying a ridiculous price.

Also implied in this recovery, is that for capillary cells to be effective in returning the interstitial space to its former glory, it must systematically retake all of the feedback loop cross talk signals that were hijacked from them by chronic inflammation. This usurping of chronic inflammatory control of the interstitial space takes time as different disease venues feedback loops must be disassembled. In addition, the disassembling may be incomplete as damaged capillary cell DNA will not afford a complete recovery of outer membrane receptors, infrastructure or mitochondrial volumes. In this scenario, a stalemate truce may occur between the forces of chronic inflammation and the capillary cell and allied forces. Implied in this détente, it the possibility that chronic inflammation can come back to preeminence if vascular inflammatory free radical fuel once again increases.

The capillary cell reverse coupe is completed when there is a complete restoration of feedback loop crosstalk with their allied interstitial space partners. This means that immune arsenal trafficked into the interstitial space is once again choreographed to a specific purpose and mesenchymal cells have been redirected to facilitate that purpose. This capillary cell reverse coupe is difficult and now without risk as excessive DNA damage may produce too much baggage for effective recovery. For this reason, "an early ounce of chronic inflammatory prevention is worth much more than a pound of cure".

What Composes an Ounce of Prevention?

For best results, start by reading a detailed discussion about prevention in my recently published books *Rejuvenation!* and *Hazing Aging*. While it may take time and there may be failures to make certain transitions towards prevention, the outcomes are worth it. There is no price on feeling your best. To make the capillary cell hum, make these habits part of an ounce of prevention:

- *Exercise* 30-35 minutes daily, preferably using a 2:1 ratio of intensive aerobic interval training with weight training. If over 35, and with preexisting medical conditions, the intensity of exercise should get a pass from your health care provider. Getting a personal trainer to help with the details may also be wise. In those fit enough, rigorous interval training is best but will need periodic tweaking to incentivize performance. Aging coefficients based on maximum exercise capacity from a stress test, which I have discussed in *Rejuvenation!* and *Hazing Aging,* can be used as a tool to estimate the capacity to exercise, a safe exercise prescription, and a gauge to physical aging. If over age 50, complement aerobic exercise and weight training with a few minutes of *balancing* and *stretching*. If you develop nagging excessive fatigue, shortness of breath or chest pains with any exercise program, see your health care provider.
- *Mediterranean or DASH* type diets (see glossary), accenting *whole food- plant based cruciferous vegetables* and a near complete elimination of simple sugars, trans-fats, processed and canned foods, and nitrosamine laced red and processed meats. When in doubt, reduce diary and white flour gluten based products (bread, pasta, crackers, potato chips, cereals, yogurt, milk, ice cream). They usually contain large amounts of hidden sugars, trans-fats, or salt.
- Other beneficial dietary add-ons include virgin cold pressed olive oil, beans, mixed preferably non- roasted and unsalted nuts, avocados, and wild fatty fish such as salmon or tuna. Organic green teas and coffee supplement water drinking and an ounce of dark chocolate (70% cocoa) daily can also be beneficial. Keep alcohol to a minimum. A couple of daily handfuls of berries, including blue, black and straw berries are the preferred fruit.
- Use of supplements and medicines that are age and diagnosis appropriate. These treatments will augment deficiency states and potentially lessen the risk of different diseases that include cancer, systemic infections, heart attacks and strokes.
- Anticipate and mitigate stress, which are situations that cause protracted anxiety or worry. Stress is mitigated by identifying and eliminating stressors. This could involve changing jobs, lessoning financial obligations or dropping certain friends or even spouses.
- An attempt at 7 hours of continuous nightly sleep, preferably without prescription drugs. Interventions include non- drug management of insomnia, improved sleep hygiene, treatment of apnea and reducing trips to the bathroom.
- Behaviors that nurture a positive social context are important. This would include for many a spiritual connection.
- Eliminate all addicting drugs, sugars and tobacco. Addictions can gateway other addictions. Alcohol, even in moderation, can reduce muscle and nerve performance while increasing pain and tremors, which compound with aging.

- Eliminate or mitigate toxic exposures from air pollutants, noxious gases, solvents, pesticides, hormones, aluminum, lead, asbestos, mercury, etc. Unfortunately, this includes most tap water, some farm produce, certain meats and poultry, and in some instances the fish we eat or the air we breathe.

When making adjustments there will be fails. The important point is to stop the behavior or choice before it metastasizes to cause collateral damage. Poor choices can cascade more poor choices which will lead to disease. Making good choices should spread to how we socialize, spend leisure time or even how we dally in front of a computer, smart phone or television. Too much television or social media will subliminally induce bad choices.

Good choices will also require a shift towards preparing more meals at home using freshly picked herbs and vegetables. I mean less eating in restaurants or picking up prepackaged food to eat on the run.

Daily exercise must be guarded as sacrosanct, but at times different aches and pains will require an exercise plan B. Don't let exercise muscle or joint pain deter consistency, but find ways to work around a nagging ailment. When in doubt consult your health care provider or trainer about alternative exercise.

Other age appropriate interventions include:

- Correcting vitamin and antioxidant deficiency states that become more common in those over 50 years of age and include treatment of thyroid deficiency, anemia and supplementing with CoQ10, vitamin D, magnesium, B vitamins, and omega three oils which become deficient with aging. Adding in fresh herbs, and turmeric, among others, will boost cellular function.
- Regular periodontal assessment and teeth cleaning.
- Focused attention to inherited genetic diseases and countering them with pre-emptive behavioral, and in some cases, medicinal treatments.
- Basic vaccines that include flu and pneumonia shots, colonoscopy, and age appropriate prostate screening and mammograms.

Chain Reactions: How Cells Mobilize Intent

The execution of optimal interstitial space homeostasis requires a series of *chain reactions* between capillary cell organelles, their outer membranes and mitochondria, as well as with other cells within the interstitial space, blood plasma, or downstream. If choreographed correctly chain reactions provide momentum to a purposed intent of optimal interstitial space sanitation and a nurtured and revitalized end organ.

When the capillary cell dance is blocked, chronic interstitial space inflammation progresses through feedback loop signaling that facilitates *pro-inflammatory chain reactions*. Proinflammatory chain reactions do the opposite of capillary choreography. They stoke inflammatory momentum, are fueled by vascular inflammatory free radicals, and perpetuate the organization of the inflammatory matrix, anti-organ, and disease venues. As these different proinflammatory venues mature, they unmask additional proinflammatory chain reactions that can include those originating from cancer cells, infectious agents, basement membrane thickening, plaque or autoimmune complexes. In this manner, proinflammatory chain reactions increase disease venue while accelerating end organ declines. When these disease venues are triggered in one end organ, they trigger additional proinflammatory chain reactions to involve capillaries and end organs elsewhere. Proinflammatory chain reactions will cause and affect all cells to eventually attempt counter adjustments.

Proinflammatory chain reactions block the capillary cell dance. They are fueled by vascular inflammatory free radicals and can be caused by any element to the immune arsenal. They can expand from misplaced or misguided sets of cytokines, lymphocytes, immunoglobulins, clotting factors or platelets. Momentum is created when a misguided cytokine attaches to a membrane surface and signals a misguided message which is then sent to a white blood cell platelet or immunoglobulin with misguided information. These cells, proteins and enzymes act on the false information to facilitate even more false signaling. The downhill snowball effect of a mistake prone proinflammatory momentum has been initiated.

Blocking proinflammatory chain reactions by eliminating their fuel will reduce their spread. As vascular inflammatory fuel decreases, the enabled capillary cell dance will resurrect trafficking choreography into the interstitial space thereby blocking the proinflammatory chain reaction by assembling an anti-inflammatory chain reaction. As interstitial space hygiene improves, disease venues go into hibernation. The effect that anti-inflammatory chain reactions have on restoring the interstitial space is called anti-inflammatory *pleotropism*. This means that the uncoupling of chronic inflammatory chain reactions within the interstitial space eliminates a broad spectrum of potential disease venues. As proinflammatory momentum unwinds cancer cells, infectious agents, and clotting biases attempt to seek refuge in obscure corners of the interstitial space. As this is occurring the end organ enjoys a renaissance return of function.

As proinflammatory momentum defervesces, their elimination may be incomplete and disease venues my still require treatment. Adding back aspirin, metformin, ACE inhibitors or statins (see *Hazing Aging* or *Rejuvenation! I Universe 2015, 2017*) may be required as well as other interventions. As proinflammatory chain reactions are subverted, aging dynamics improve as does pain and fatigue. All causes of age related declines decrease or are postponed and include strokes, heart attacks, different cancers, disabling arthritis, dementias and different lung, kidney and liver diseases.

Chain reactions, pro or anti-inflammatory, comes down to who controls interstitial space. Eliminating vascular inflammatory free radical fuel pushes the odds favoring anti-inflammatory pleotropism. *Preempt to prevent.*

CHAPTER 6

PERMEABILITY MECHANICS OF TRAFFICKING

Introducing Permeability Mechanics

Persistent migration of vascular inflammatory free radical fuel into interstitial spaces and on endothelial –capillary cell basement membranes is the calling card for our innate immune arsenal to come towards them. How and when they get there defines permeability mechanics. Capillary and endothelial cells choreograph immune arsenal to come into the interstitial space to remove the offending molecule, toxin, metabolite, particle or gas. Capillary outer membrane glycocalyx and continuous outer membrane receptors, are reconfigured to enable specific immune arsenal attachments from blood plasma. They proceed to enter the staging area of the interstitial space, seek the offending molecule, bind to it, and then release their own set of cytokines to other immune arsenal, capillary and mesenchymal cells to further accomplish removal of the offending agent. The entire process is choreographed when capillary cells enable the arrival of immune arsenal and the removal of breach suspects.

If vascular free radicals fester within the interstitial space, things change. Acting as chronic inflammatory fuel, they attract immune arsenal, freeze capillary mitochondrial combustion, compromise outer membrane receptors to induce a proinflammatory tsunami of chain reactions that shift the interstitial spaces to dark outcomes.

The gutted capillary cell, robbed of infrastructure, competent DNA, mitochondrial volumes and outer membrane receptors loses its capacity to choreograph as well as ability to feedback loop signal to its partners. The interstitial space caves to a chronic inflammatory set of cytokine feedback loops and agendas.

When feedback loops relationships within the interstitial space change hands, wayward trafficked immune arsenal will actively convert mesenchymal cells to the chronic inflammatory cause. The new prerogative is to hijack the disabled capillary cell outer membranes and use them to traffic a new order within the interstitial space. Now, the newly arriving immune arsenal will be influenced to support a different purpose which is to promote disease venues. The game plan of using the body's own immune arsenal to exploit disease venues, through the zombied capillary cell, and at the expense of the true end organ, has been set in place. This pattern defines the executive operational mechanics of chronic inflammation.

Let's summarize the transition of interstitial space from light to darkness.

- Vascular inflammatory free radicals penetrate and impinge the interstitial space in alarming numbers and diversity. They attach to membrane surfaces, subvert membrane function and attract immune arsenal towards them.
- Capillary cell outer membrane permeability persistently increases to immune arsenal migration into the interstitial space.
- Their mitochondrial combustion gets stuck in energy to support active transport of immune arsenal.
- Superoxide exhaust accumulates within the capillary cell and denatures nuclear DNA
- From combinations of denatured DNA and blocked protein synthesis of poorly coded proteins, capillary cell infrastructure falls apart.
- Capillary cell mitochondrial volumes decrease as does outer membrane receptors, voltage gradients and pore diversity known as pseudocapillarization.
- A non- purposed mistake prone immune arsenal enters the interstitial space.
- They create their own cytokine feedback loop signaling system that overrides and then hijacks those from the capillary cell.
- As feedback loop momentum shifts purpose, from capillary cell choreography to chronic inflammatory chaos, mesenchymal cells are converted.
- The interstitial space becomes hostile to the true end organ as disease venues involving scarring, thrombosis, cancer, infections and autoimmune diseases proliferate.
- The inflammatory process relies on vascular inflammatory free radicals to fuel and expand operations to eventually take down the end organ.

Different inflammatory breaches sequence different sets of immune arsenal. In many instances, where breach comes from a particle, infectious agent, or some other rogue molecule, the initial choreographed response by capillary cells involves receptor attachment of *neutrophil white blood* cells. After neutrophils enter the interstitial space staging area, they attach and spray their granules. The sprayed granules begin the process of breach containment while also acting as a signaling force back to capillary cell outer membranes and mesenchymal cells for additional immune arsenal reinforcements. The signal will either call for additional neutrophil back-up or to send in the next wave of attack. This wave would include different sets of cytokines as well as *B and T lymphocytes.* In this phase, the process of *breach elimination and clean up* begins. As each step nears completion, the same signaling pattern occurs at the capillary cell outer membranes. The remaining immune arsenal at the breach site, collectively signal the capillary cell outer membranes to choreograph the next step, until the breach is removed and the interstitial space is made whole.

When completed, capillary cell outer membranes are signaled from what immune arsenal remains at the staging area to reduce trafficking into the interstitial space. This shifts outer membrane permeability as capillary cells divest unneeded energy and calcium ions back to their mitochondria. As capillary cell outer membrane reconfigures the cell from oval to flat, outer membrane receptors go into hiding within the membrane infrastructure. As energy and calcium ions re- accumulate within the mitochondria, they feedback loop a switch in combustion form energy to nitric oxide. Capillary and endothelial cells then shift purpose.

When chronic inflammation changes the feedback loop equation within the interstitial space, trafficking of neutrophils, B and T lymphocytes and cytokines is disrupted. These different cells are enabled to enter the interstitial space staging area at the wrong place and time. These mismatches collectively induce signaling feedback loops to capillary and mesenchymal cells that confuse purpose and cloud intent. It increases the likelihood that inflammatory breach will not be removed and perhaps even expanded. The aggregate momentum of these aberrant signals will promote chronic inflammatory expansion and block the capillary cell dance.

The expanding feedback loop deception involves trafficking into the interstitial space, of not only white blood cells, but also cytokines, platelets, immunoglobulins, clotting factors and other inflammatory proteins. It is in this context that proinflammatory momentum takes over the interstitial space as its communication links replace those of disabled capillary cells.

Second line inflammatory mediators, or innate immune arsenal, are derived from the liver, lymph tissue, spleen or bone marrow. In some cases, as with cytokines, they can originate from a variety of different cells, including capillary, mesenchymal and end organ cells, and can elicit different effects depending on whom, when and where they are released. This implies that cascading an effective immune response into an interstitial space involves a sophisticated "lock and key system" that creates momentum as well as fostering appropriate steps in processing an immune response. These feedback loop signals build and stack on each other as one lock and key opens the next door of the immune response. When properly choreographed by capillary cells, the immune response to inflammatory breach is unveiled like a classic masterpiece. When the lock and keys become desynchronized, immune trafficking by capillary cells becomes mistake prone and suboptimal to breach elimination. Eventually inflammatory breach gets the upper hand. The more that immune arsenal trafficking gets scrambled, the worse things become for the end organ.

The Trafficking Death March

Vascular inflammatory free radical fuel largely determines how well the capillary cell choreography operates. A small trickling of vascular inflammatory free radicals entering the interstitial space can usually be disposed of without disrupting interstitial space homeostasis. Larger volumes, particularly if diversified and persistent over time, are a much different story. In this setting, proinflammatory cascades within interstitial spaces become inevitable.

What are the mechanics of an interstitial space coupe? It begins with free radical impingement within interstitial spaces, progresses with wayward white blood cells migration into the staging area, and is then perpetuated by the release of misguided cytokines (lymphokines) which further disrupt inflammatory breach containment and elimination. This proinflammatory momentum chain reacts, forms its own feedback loop momentum, hijacks the disabled capillary cell outer membranes, and proceeds to enable more rebel immune arsenal entry into the interstitial space as progressive chronic inflammation consolidates and begins processing disease venues. This defines the trafficking death march. As anti-organ disease venues escalate the true end organ shrinks in stature.

Disease venues are often shaped by the type of rogue immune arsenal assemblage within the interstitial space, the dependency of end organ function on oxygen, and genetic predisposition. Once there is sufficient capillary cell capitulation, and depending on these three variables, disease venues will populate the interstitial space and form different levels of scarring, thrombosis, cancer, infections or autoimmune diseases. As cancer cells or infectious agents populate the interstitial space, they can construct their own defense-support systems using combinations of infiltrated immune arsenal, converted mesenchymal cells and imported growth factors. As they advance the true end organ becomes increasingly marginalized. The coupe by chronic inflammation becomes a feedback loop exchange of rogue cytokine signals from the wrong cell at the wrong time and place to cause immune interstitial space anarchy. It is through immune anarchy that the interstitial space picks its poison. Short of removing vascular free radical fuel, there is no capillary cell escape clause. The only way out of this death trap is for a capillary cell reenactment of their dance.

Choreography

For purposeful immune arsenal trafficking into the interstitial space, capillary cell outer membranes must be capable of sequencing their arrival through fluxing adjustments to permeability, which is known as capillary cell *choreography*. Sequencing of immune arsenal into interstitial spaces requires intricate coordination of capillary cell outer membrane protein kinase on-off switches, receptor exposures, gap junction widening, fluxing voltage gradients, a diverse pore system, vesicle and transport channels, and a generous supply of energy and calcium ions from mitochondria. The quality assurance of choreography quality is dependent on a healthy pivot of outer membrane permeability so as to signal mitochondria to swing combustion to nitric oxide. Doing so enables replacement of worn out outer membrane receptors and enzymes, augmenting mitochondrial volumes and restoring capillary cell infrastructure. The swing in combustion also helps to keep superoxide exhaust damage to a minimum while helping to restore depleted antioxidant reserves. The permeability pivot and swing in mitochondrial combustion implies that effective capillary cell choreography must be successful in eliminating inflammatory breach.

The crux of well -organized capillary cell choreography is its capacity to expose exact sets of outer membrane receptors to attach a precise immune arsenal that will be focused on eliminating inflammatory breach. Rotation ensures specific sequencing of white blood cells, platelets and immunoglobulins which attack and release cytokines that participate in the lock and key momentum of eventual breach removal. The released cytokines tie in mesenchymal cell responses as well as giving further instructions to capillary cells about what else should be brought into the staging area to facilitate breach elimination. The precision and pace of outer membrane receptor exposures, becomes dependent on what comes before it. If the cytokine feedback loop signals are crisp the receptor exposures will be more definitive in delivering the correct immune response. Outer membrane receptor exposures are not only dependent on cytokine signals but also on the capacity of outer membrane infrastructure. In this manner, how well the outer membranes bend and twist will determine how exact receptor exposures will become.

Successful capillary cell outer membrane choreography results in a purposeful mosaic of carefully sequenced and targeted immune arsenal into the interstitial space staging area. When successful, it will contain and eliminate any inflammatory breach. The end result is restoration of interstitial space homeostasis, and a rigorous downshift of capillary cell outer membrane fluxed permeability to trafficked immune arsenal. Capillary cell choreography is the essential piece to optimal interstitial space homeostasis and end organ viability.

Nitric Oxide: The Gas of Rejuvenation or Cyanide Poisoning

Healthy capillary cell outer membrane fluxing of permeability and mitochondrial swinging of combustion facilitates the dual purpose maintenance of interstitial space sanitation while nurturing oxygen and nutrient supply to the end organ. When capillary cell nitric oxide combustion is signaled, it becomes the rejuvenating capillary cell gas of repair and replacement, while through outer membrane and mitochondrial feedback loop signals, paces similar effects to its interstitial space allies. As such nitric oxide combustion becomes a quality assurance buffer. When coupled with reductions in vascular inflammatory free radicals and a rigorous capillary cell dance, it fuels anti-aging, disease resistance. Remissions in fatigue and pain are not far behind.

Whether capillary cell mitochondria are combusting energy or nitric oxide, the molecular *hub* of combustion is *acetyl coenzyme A (acetyl CoA)*. Acetyl CoA is produced the breakdown of *pyruvate, fatty acids and ketone bodies*. When energy combustion is required, as occurs with the active transport of immune arsenal, acetyl CoA is looped into the *Krebs cycle*. On the other hand, when mitochondria swing combustion to nitric oxide, acetyl CoA is *shuttled* to nearby ribosomes and rough endoplasmic reticulum in the cytoplasm where it is utilized to manufacture proteins for repair or replacement of capillary cell infrastructure. The protein synthesis from nitric oxide combustion quality assures *replacement* of outer membrane receptors while also regenerating mitochondrial volumes. It also causes *activation of telomerase* the enzyme that replaces the telomere cap, which protects nuclear DNA from free radical cross linkage. Without the repair and replacement of infrastructure the capillary cell will morph into a passive and easily manipulated cell.

The nitric oxide gas can also diffuse through capillary outer membranes and increase relaxation of adjacent arteriole smooth muscle. This causes an increase in blood flow towards the capillary bed.

In this manner, capillary cells increase oxygenated blood flow to the end organ. By allowing the end organ's mitochondria greater access to oxygen, it signals for more energy combustion, which improves end organ function.

When capillary mitochondria get stuck in energy combustion, as when the interstitial space is gripped by chronic inflammation, the excessive superoxide exhaust, chain reacts damage to infrastructure and DNA. In the end organ, this mitochondrial feedback loop causes their mitochondria to get stuck in nitric oxide combustion, which causes the toxic buildup of hydroxynitriles, the first cousin to cyanide gas. Neither superoxide nor cyanide works out very well for either cell's infrastructure or DNA. Mitochondrial sticking chain reacts both capillary and end organ futility and keys chronic inflammatory interstitial space progression.

Immune Arsenal: Pro or Anti-Inflammatory or Both

The immune arsenal that compose secondary inflammatory mediators are like the skin of a salamander. Its skin can change color based on prevailing conditions within its environment. Immune arsenal can also change allegiance within interstitial spaces based on who or what is signaling them. Signaling circumstances, based on prevailing conditions within the interstitial space, will either reduce or expand inflammatory responses, to eliminate or perpetuate an interstitial space inflammatory breach.

An example of this is found in nitric oxide (NO). When NO is combusted by capillary cell mitochondria, it signals a decrease in outer membrane permeability, a reversal of inflammatory momentum within the interstitial space and a rejuvenation of capillary cell infrastructure while nurturing improvements to end organ function. On the other hand, when NO is released from white blood cells within the interstitial space, it can have an opposite effect of *expanding additional inflammation*. This means, that when nitric oxide is released from interstitial space white blood cells, it has the opposite effect than when it is produced in capillary cells. When inflammation is expanded by white blood cell release of nitric oxide, it chains reacts release of proinflammatory growth factors and perpetuates increases in capillary cell outer membrane immune arsenal trafficking.

Thus nitric oxide release by different cells in different places can cause a different mosaic of effects. With the proinflammatory biases that occur with chronic inflammation, it increases the likelihood of rebel white blood cells within the interstitial space will release more nitric oxide which will perpetuate interstitial space inflammation while also blocking nitric oxide production from involved capillary cells.

Making anti-inflammatory lifestyle adjustments, that decrease vascular inflammatory free radical fuel within interstitial spaces, becomes the critical first step in re –establishing the capillary cell dance. This shifts feedback loop momentum away from rebel interstitial space white blood cells and towards capillary cell choreography. In the case of nitric oxide, it means capillary cells reestablishing control of nitric oxide production while limiting the effects of white cell generated nitric oxide. When this occurs, momentum switches direction towards restoring interstitial space sanitation.

Nitric oxide is just one of several different cytokines like molecules that can be both pro or anti-inflammatory depending on who releases them. It comes back to how well capillary cells are choreographing.

A Closer Look at Immune Arsenal

The table below represents a partial list of human immune arsenal, also referred to as second-line inflammatory mediators. As with the example of nitric oxide, immune arsenal can either expand or contract inflammation within interstitial spaces based on who or what is signaling them. Containing or eliminating interstitial space inflammatory breach, facilitates capillary cell outer membrane choreography, whereas a smoldering chronic inflammatory interstitial space does the opposite. Table 2 represents a sampling of commonly known immune arsenal. In the context of capillary cell choreography, expanding the inflammatory response is beneficial to breach elimination. When inflammatory mediators are released from rebel white blood cells or elsewhere, expanding the inflammatory response promotes more destructive inflammation.

TABLE 2-Examples of Inflammatory Mediators that Expand Inflammation

Inflammatory Mediator Mechanics of Induction

- Lymphocytes (B and T cells) Promotes proliferation of an immune response
- Effector and memory T cells Promotes proliferation of an immune response
- Neutrophils Promotes proliferation of an immune response
- Macrophages/foam cells Promotes proliferation of an immune response
- Complement system Stimulates immune inflammation
- Cytokines (ex. IL-6) Can be chemokines, interferons, or tumor necrosis factor
- C Reactive Protein (also HSCRP) Made in the liver, increases IL-6,macrophages
- PAR 1-2 protease activated receptors Modulates immune inflammation
- Immunoglobulins Stimulates immune inflammation
- Leukotrienes Stimulates immune inflammation
- Histamine Stimulates immune inflammation
- Prostaglandins Stimulates immune inflammation
- PAI-1 (Serpin E-1) Inhibits t-PA, increases thrombosis
- Thromboxane A-2 Platelet generated vasoconstrictor/pro- coagulant
- Serum amyloid A lipoproteins Liver produced, stimulates immune inflammation
- Fibrinogen Liver produced, pro coagulant
- VEGF (endothelial cell growth factor) Stimulates immune inflammation

- Growth factors Stimulates immune inflammation
- Thrombin Stimulate immune inflammation
- Bradykinin-Kallikreins Stimulates immune inflammation
- Nitric oxide Released from WBCs, stimulates immune inflammation

The list is not all-inclusive, nor is the mechanics of immune modulation described in detail. What is important is that immune arsenal expansion of inflammation with interstitial spaces can work for good or for darker purposes. If the capillary cell is choreographing they become anti –inflammatory. If the inflammatory matrix or anti-organ controls the interstitial space, they become pro-inflammatory. This means our own immune arsenal will actually cause self-destruction within interstitial spaces depending on who they take their cues from.

The above list also does not do justice to the different nuanced effects of family members within a given set of immune arsenal. In other words, regardless of who is in charge of the interstitial space, different family members within a given immune arsenal family will nuance different inflammatory effects which further mosaic the inflammatory response as they create an elaborate lock and key checks and balances system. Inflammatory expansion is nuanced based on different *contexts*.

As an example a specific growth factor will have a different effect based on *what member* within the family of growth factors is being produced, by *what cell* it is being produced from, and *where* the production is occurring. Like the example of nitric oxide, a given growth factor released by a capillary cell will have a decidedly different effect than when produced by a white blood cell in the interstitial space. When capillary cells are controlling the context of growth factor release, their effects will contain and eliminate inflammatory breach and support the end organ. On the other hand, when growth factors are being released by rogue white blood cells, there is no precise choreography. Instead, proinflammatory momentum causes growth factors to be released for the wrong reasons thereby expanding chronic inflammation without eliminating the interstitial space inflammatory breach.

With chronic inflammation, the proinflammatory context within interstitial spaces of released growth factors or any other cytokine being released by rebel white blood cells is driven by *randomness, contributes to more immune mistakes and eventually supports anti-organ disease venues.*

The Pitch Battle for Interstitial Space Control

At any given moment within the interstitial spaces of end organs, there is a pitch battle between forces that expand inflammation randomly and those that expand it with intent to eliminate breach. Capillary cell outer membranes are in a push and pull of permeability adjustments that struggle to maintain sequenced choreography. At any given moment they are provided cytokine intelligence to their outer membrane surfaces that facilitates breach removal or expansion. As more rebel white blood cells find their way into the interstitial space, not only are capillary cell mitochondria overheating from excessive energy combustion, their outer membranes are getting cytokine feedback that betrays inflammatory breach removal. In this case, the pitch battle favors evolving chronic inflammation.

The reverse occurs if vascular inflammatory free radical fuel is reduced. In this case, inflammatory momentum favors capillary cell choreography and inflammatory breach removal from the interstitial space.

This capacity to *flux outer membrane permeability* back and forth forms the basis for effective capillary cell choreography, rejuvenation and interstitial space homeostasis. It is blocked by vascular inflammatory free radicals and progressive chronic inflammatory momentum within the interstitial space.

Chronic inflammation cascades many things, but its first order of business it provide enough cytokine feedback loop signaling back to capillary cell membranes to blur capillary cell clarity of interstitial space purpose. This cytokine smoke screen, is initially induced by abundant vascular inflammatory free radicals within the interstitial space, but takes on a life of its own as rebel white blood cells and other ineffective immune arsenal come into the interstitial space and propagate false signals. This rogue feedback loop assault chain reacts even more immune arsenal errors by capillary cell outer membranes entering the interstitial space. The capillary cell eventually degrades from the inside out on the basis of mitochondrial overheating and superoxide toxicity.

Inflammatory Mediators that Bias Contraction of Inflammation

Table three below, demonstrates a group of secondary inflammatory mediators that bias contraction of the inflammatory response. Many of these mediators, such as macrophages, different cytokines and T cells, can also expand inflammation. Therefore, expansion or contraction of inflammation depends on context and who is in control of the interstitial space. Therefore, the breakdown of immune arsenal into expanders and contractors of inflammation would appear arbitrary as so much rides on what controls the interstitial space.

In the table, when I reference PPARs, the sirtuin family, CAMP (cyclic adenosine monophosphate), S1P and nitric oxide, I am referring to effects produced when their release or activation comes from endothelia. In the grand scheme, when sequenced properly, these mediators provide momentum for the feedback loop swing of endothelial mitochondrial combustion to nitric oxide. This becomes vital for capillary cell repair and replacement of infrastructure to avoid loss of outer membrane receptors or mitochondrial volumes.

When properly choreographed, many of these inflammatory mediators in the table below contract inflammation by detailing interstitial space *elimination* and *clean-up* of inflammatory debris. These same inflammatory mediators, when under the influence of rebel immune arsenal within the interstitial space, can act as immune suppressants and block recognition of bacteria, viruses or cancer cells.

In addition, for a given inflammatory context, different family members of say the sirtuin group, will nuance different effects on capillary cell outer membranes that can range from reducing to increasing permeability to trafficked immune arsenal. Thus when sirtuin family members are released for the wrong reasons, they will chain react misguided trafficking responses into the interstitial space. This eventually could lead to ineffective recognition of foreign invaders or cancer cells.

TABLE Three- Inflammatory Mediators that Bias Inflammatory Contraction

- Macrophages Mop up-swallow/digest/eliminate inflammatory debris
- Cytokines Participate in free radical –invader clean-up
- T cells Inhibits immune response after free radical containment
- PPARS (peroxisome activator receptor) Improves insulin sensitivity, glucose metabolism
- Sirtuins blunt mitochondrial ATP/calcium ion release
- Prostacyclin (PGI-2) Platelet inhibitor, arterial vasodilator
- C-AMP(cyclic adenosine monophosphate) smooth muscle vasodilator, activates PKA
- Adiponectin from fat cells Suppresses adhesion, modulates immune response
- HDL cholesterol Inhibits conversion of LDL to OX LDL (very inflammatory)
- Angiopoietin 1 (ANG-1) Decreases capillary cell membrane permeability
- S1P Decreases capillary cell membrane permeability
- Sphingosine Decreases endothelial cell permeability
- Albumin Stabilizes capillary cell outer membrane permeability
- Nitric oxide Released from capillaries, decreases membrane permeability
- Interleukin 10 Inhibits activation of T lymphocytes and monocytes

Successful trafficking of inflammatory mediators into interstitial spaces depends on precise capillary cell choreography. When successful, the inflammatory breach is eliminated and capillary cells are enabled to downshift outer membrane permeability and swing mitochondrial combustion. This becomes the key homeostasis piece to managing their own vitality, that of the interstitial space and the end organ.

When capillary cell basement membranes are being harmed by excessive free radicals, this chain reacts a blocked pivot and swing dance. As this occurs, signals of interstitial space intent become blurred and eventually replaced by rebel signals. As purpose is blurred, immune arsenal expanders might contract and contractors expand as entering interstitial space immune arsenal gets and increasingly convoluted set of signals. Disease venues within the interstitial space become inevitableoutcomes.

CHAPTER 7

THE CONSOLIDATION OF CHRONIC INTERSTITIAL SPACE INFLAMMATION

An Introduction

Brace yourself. At this juncture, for those not proficient in the biological sciences, you must become familiar with a new language. I will keep this dialogue as simple as I can so as to not lose credibility. Language can be a powerful tool. Embrace the biological language like you might French, Russian or Spanish and a deeper understanding will occur. If you keep one finger pinned to the glossary of terms found in the back of the book, context and meaning will become evident.

To summarize, chronic inflammation within end organ interstitial spaces is birthed by vascular inflammatory free radicals entering and impinging interstitial spaces and endothelial/capillary cell basement membrane surfaces. Its festering sends our own immune arsenal towards them in attempts to contain and eliminate them. If it fails, the chronic pestering effect of free radical impingement blocks the capillary cell pivot and swing dance and keeps their mitochondria combusting energy to support active transport. This increases superoxide free radical buildup, damages membrane infrastructure and both nuclear and mitochondrial DNA, and prevents capillary cells from nitric oxide driven rejuvenation. As capillary cells lose their effectiveness to take care of themselves, choreograph immune arsenal and respond to end organ requirements, they enable a more random funneling of immune arsenal into the interstitial space, which over time replaces the weakened capillary cell feedback loops with their own brand. Once signaling feedback loop have been hijacked, the equivalent of an interstitial space coupe has occurred, that has replaced capillary cell choreography and response to end organ functional requirements with an increasingly hostile feedback loop system that *perpetuates* disease venues while *marginalizing* the end organ. It turns out the stemming and pacing of the capillary cell dance makes or breaks the capillary cell itself and all the interstitial space infrastructure including the end organ. With all this in mind, let us look at outcomes to chronic interstitial space inflammation.

Chronic Shear Inflammation, Basement Membrane Thickening and Hypertension

Hypertension is defined as a persistent increase in the conduit pressures within arterial lumens and is universally recognized when arm cuff blood pressures meet or exceed 140/90 mmHg. Implied in hypertension is the diminution of endothelial responsiveness to dilate or constrict blood vessel lumens due to the buildup of chronic inflammatory residues on basement membranes. Hypertension is associated with basement membrane thickening throughout the vascular tree but carries particular risk to bifurcating lumens where a larger vessel divides into two smaller ones. The primary outcome to basement membrane thickening and the corresponding increase in luminal pressures is increased *shear stress.*

Shear inflammation feeds on itself, as increases in intraluminal pressures create more shear inflammation and injury to endothelial lumen surfaces. The result is a progressive thickening of abluminal endothelial basement membranes as their luminal glycocalyx thins. The progression disrupts endothelial cell homeostasis and makes them less capable in managing the interstitial space or responding to their end organ. In the case of larger arterial vessels, they decrease responsiveness to the smooth muscle cells that live them. Although it is not known at what blood pressure shear injury commences, current theory suggests that hypertensive injury to large vessel membrane surfaces begins at blood pressures above 120/85 mmHg with injury accelerating as blood pressures increase.

Since hypertension is birthed by vascular inflammatory free radical seeding of endothelial basement membranes, it becomes an early and sensitive clinical indicator of vascular free radical impingement to basement membrane surfaces. The free radicals can come from a variety of different sources, but most commonly include *AGEs (advanced glycation end products)* from elevated blood sugars, excessive salt ingestion, numerous inhaled tobacco free radicals, the ingestion of certain drugs and alcohol, or the accumulation of circulating small *particle LDL cholesterol, lipoprotein (a), non HDL cholesterols, or homocysteine.* It can also occur from excessive circulating stress hormones that increase from sleep deprivation, sleep apneas, stress or chronic illness.

The persistence of these free radical impingements to basement membranes, plumes an immune arsenal response which then thickens the membrane surfaces over time. As basement membranes thicken, the endothelial cell loses capacity to effectively communicate with the smooth muscle cells that surround them. This blocked communication between endothelial cell and smooth muscle creates the opening for hypertension. Free radical impingement on basement membranes leading to hypertension is associated with a blocked pivot and swing dance with mitochondrial combustion getting stuck in energy. This eventually makes the endothelium even less capable in managing blood vessel lumen mechanics. Instead, lumen walls progressively stiffen and become much less responsive to adjustment. The progression of basement membrane thickening to an obstructive plaque becomes a disease venue within the interstitial space of a large arterial vessel that can lead to compromised blood flow to upstream end organs. Numerous adverse outcomes will result from this potentially catastrophic progression.

Of the numerous adverse chain reaction that occur with hypertension, a major development involves feedback loops to liver, kidney and lung that trigger increases in circulating *angiotensin II*. Angiotensin II and similar hormones are activated by increases in arterial lumen pressures coupled with less oxygen delivery to liver, kidney and lung. The release and activation of angiotensin II actually increases blood pressure further by causing large vessel arterial smooth muscles to contract, which makes hypertension even worse. This misread has huge ramifications to hypertensive related complications involving several end organs.

Hypertension does much of its basement membrane and glycocalyx inflammatory damage in stealth, with symptoms emerging only after pressures are substantially elevated, or end organs compromised from reduced blood flows. When large arterial vessel basement membrane thickening matures it often culminates in the development of obstructive plaque. Obstructive plaque contains a mixture of vascular inflammatory free radicals, white blood cells, platelets, clotting factors and calcium. As it grows on basement membranes, its weight impinges lumen diameters to obstruct and eventually slow the flow of blood through the impingement. This impingement becomes at risk for a clot related occlusion. The risk for vascular events to upstream end organs usually begins to escalate when large vessel lumens have been narrowed by 70%, with thrombosis risks leading to a vascular occlusion and blood flow cutoff occurring when the obstructive plaque impinges 90% of the lumen orifice. It stands to reason that preventing and treating elevated blood pressure by reducing vascular inflammatory free radicals becomes central to limiting end organ collateral damage.

Double Whammy Effect

The *double whammy effect* describes the predicament where capillary cells often caught in the middle of end organ demands for more oxygen and downstream endothelia not being able to deliver the necessary blood volumes to accommodate the demand. The double whammy comes from the effects of vascular inflammatory free radicals that thicken basement membranes up and down the arterial tree from the largest of vessels to the smallest of capillaries. It turns out that this thickening limits the capacity of larger vessels to respond to increased demands upstream for oxygen and the capillaries upstream have a tougher time executing oxygen delivery through their basement membranes to eventually find its way to end organ outer membranes. The combination of decreased on demand oxygen delivery and decreased capacity to diffuse the gas through their basement membranes due to its thickness, defines double whammy. The double whammy causes a double hit on end organ function, as it is left often holding the bag of requiring more on demand oxygen to optimally function but not getting it. In oxygen sensitive end organs such as heart or brain, function deteriorates to the level of oxygen deficit. Heart muscles cannot contract as forcefully and brain cells cannot send electrical messages as deeply into the brain. Muscle and brain cells atrophy and are often replaced with filler scar tissue.

Making matters potentially worse, is how capillaries try to fix the double whammy. Capillary cells attempt resuscitation of oxygen deficits by producing growth factors, such as VEGF (vascular endothelial growth factor). This will induce capillary cells to divide and grow new capillaries but without more blood flow coming from downstream blood vessels, this becomes fruitless. Unless there is *collateral circulation* from another larger blood vessel downstream capable of redistributing regional blood to where the end organ is hypoxic, growing new capillaries will not help improve an oxygen starved end organ.

By endothelial up and won the arterial tree feeling the pinch of basement membrane thickening from vascular inflammatory free radicals, the only way to harness control of the double whammy, is to decrease them. This will offer a chance that basement membrane thickening will stall or even reverse thereby opening the gates to more blood and oxygen flow. The double whammy effect becomes the ACE in the hand for chronic inflammation. By blocking oxygen delivery to the end organ and limiting capillary cell options to manage it, double whammy sets up disease venues involving hypoxia-ischemia (strokes, heat attacks), scarring and a progressive decline in the end organs capacity to receive oxygen, in effect suffocating.

The Mechanics of Large Vessel Obstructive Plaque

When large vessel endothelial cell basement membranes thicken, from combinations of vascular inflammatory free radical and immune arsenal attachment, inflammation progress on the membrane surface to form an *obstructive plaque*. Obstructive plaque can occur anywhere in the arterial tree, but is most prone to occur where a single vessel bifurcates into two. This is because of the increase in shear that is inherent to a sudden 50% reduction in lumen diameter. As obstructive plaque matures, it gets heavy and begins to impinge on adjacent endothelial cells thereby compressing the vessel lumen. As the lumen narrows initially blood velocity through the narrowed lumen increases. As the plaque grows and obstructs further, often to reduce lumen diameters to less than 10% of normal, blood velocities through the narrowing slow. This slowing it what sets up risks for occlusion of the vessel by thrombosis, thereby cutting off oxygen supply to all vessels upstream it what can be a catastrophic event.

As soft plaque matures it often form a hard calcium cap that acts like a shell. The mature plaque can have a calcium shell and contain years of accumulated proinflammatory debris consisting of decomposed white blood cells, fibrous tissue, clotting factors, platelets, and of course vascular inflammatory free radicals. These can have origin from tobacco, LDL cholesterol, non HDL cholesterols, homocysteine, lipo (a), triglycerides and AGEs among several others.

The combination of a large calcified plaque and an increase in pressure within it, can result in plaque rupture. When obstructive plaque ruptures, it can cause a catastrophic event upstream by several mechanisms. First the affected blood vessel becomes unstable and has likely developed a hole through its endothelium meaning that blood is leaking out of the vessel lumen. Not only is this a medical emergency, but the sudden drop in blood pressures and blood flows will inevitably cause the end organ upstream to become ischemic and die.

In addition, with rupture, there is a spraying effect of inflammatory debris being sent into the lumen where it can travel upstream and become an embolus. The embolus can lodge into smaller upstream blood vessel lumens and begin processes of thrombosis leading to complete occlusion. The spraying effect might cause multiple emboli and a stuttering of devastating end organ ischemic events. None of these outcomes portend end organ viability. Other large vessel outcomes to obstructive plaque may include the development of *aneurysms* (weakened and dilated arterial wall), or *transections* (splitting) of the blood vessel where the plaque ruptured. Without properly times interventions the weakened vessel wall could eventually rupture to cause a sudden death.

The double whammy effect of progressive thickening of downstream endothelial basement membranes produces a double whammy effect that can make upstream capillary cell attempts to address hypoxia futile. The problem will only increase as long as vascular inflammatory free radicals swarm basement membranes.

The Cytokine Mechanics of Chronic Inflammatory Trafficking

How do immune arsenal message capillary outer membranes to expand inflammation within interstitial spaces? It starts with vascular inflammatory free radicals migrating and attaching to basement membrane and other surfaces within interstitial spaces. Depending on which free radicals appear, they will cause activation of cytokines, specifically those coming from early responder white blood cells, with *IL-6* (*interleukin 6*) cytokine being one of the most prolific. *When* IL-6 attaches to endothelial cell membrane surfaces it activates certain protein kinase switches, while also reducing levels of cAMP. This combination gooses endothelial and capillary cell outer membranes to increase permeability which enables additional immune arsenal arriving from blood plasma to attach to membrane newly exposed receptors. When permeability increases endothelial and capillary outer membranes *bend and twist* their infrastructure to expose different sets of *CAMs (adhesion* molecules or *receptors that include integrins, selectins and cadherins).*

When specific CAMS are exposed they enable attachment of a choreographed assemblage of white blood cells and other necessary immune arsenal in response to the inflammatory breach. Once attached by CAMS, the white blood cells can signal for additional immune arsenal attachments and/ or can be rolled to the gap junction orifice to enter the gap junction channel. Once in the channel, they are further vetted by different canals and receptors which can specify and pace what immune arsenal is allocated to the interstitial space. If not vetted through the gap junction, immune arsenal including different white blood cells they can be engulfed from outer membrane receptors into transport *vesicles* or transcellular *channels and transported* quickly to the interstitial space staging area on the abluminal side of the endothelial cell.

In addition to the cytokine IL-6, other circulating chemo proteins help facilitate an inflammatory response and help bridge endothelia and capillary cell trafficking mechanics. While IL-6 is an early responder to inflammatory breach, *MCP-1 (monocyte chemoprotein-1)* participates much later in the mechanics of breach removal. MCP-1 is a family of proteins, that when activated, nuance the elimination phase of inflammatory breach. Whereas IL-6 expands interstitial space immune arsenal, MCP-1 signals *contraction* of immune arsenal entry into the interstitial space, and becomes a critical feedback loop for the capillary cell pivot of permeability and swing of mitochondrial combustion to nitric oxide. In this fashion, MCP-1 becomes an important marker of successful breach elimination. Both IL-6 and MCP-1 are important for reestablishing interstitial space homeostasis, but with aging and chronic inflammation, IL-6 levels increase while MCP-1 levels decrease within interstitial spaces and endothelial cell outer membranes.

IL-6 and MCP-1 are two examples of inflammatory cytokines that signal pivots to inflammatory expansion or contraction. They counterbalance each other and as such become important to the mechanics of breach elimination and capillary-endothelial cells swinging combustion to nitric oxide. These two opposing cytokines, not only have an important role to play in eliminating inflammatory breach from the interstitial space, but they feedback loop back to endothelial cell outer membranes to pivot and swing their dance. When chronic inflammation establishes a foothold within the interstitial space, IL-6 levels increase relative to MCP-1, yielding biases towards a blocked endothelial- capillary cell dance, a stuck mitochondria combustion in energy, increasing superoxide damage to nuclear DNA, and a progressively disabled endothelial-capillary cell. As they zombie, signaling distortions chain react inappropriate immune arsenal into the interstitial space leading to an eventual interstitial space coupe.

Imbalances of IL-6 and MCP-1, as well as other cytokines, will up-tick chronic inflammatory risk. As immune arsenal within interstitial spaces becomes increasingly rebel, basement membranes thicken, end organ function withers and disease venue pop-ups, including hypertension, are generated. The mismatched IL-6/ MCP-1 is just one of several cytokines that can become hostile to blocking the capillary cell dance.

What surprises is how responsive hypertension can be to lifestyle choices, especially if initiated early in the process. By reducing salt, eliminating tobacco, decreasing LDL cholesterol, losing weight and exercising regularly, blood pressure resets lower to where medication is not needed. What is inferred is that to a large extent large arterial vessel stiffness, caused from basement membrane thickening, can be reversed. These low-tech lifestyle interventions not only bode well for hypertension, but for other disease venues as well.

Diabetes Mellitus

As we age we accumulate vascular inflammatory risk which are linked to vascular inflammatory free radicals, unbalanced mitochondrial combustion, and the insipid damage to nuclear DNA, brought about by either superoxide (endothelial cell) or hydroxynitrile (end organ cell) exhaust.

Included in the aging conundrum are elevations of blood sugar. Aging increases insulin resistance. We move less, carry more weight, develop atrophied skeletal muscles, eat fast food, sleep less fitfully and are prone to more anxiety and worry. All of these behaviors increase insulin resistance. In some cases, blood sugars will elevate to full blown diabetes.

As blood sugars increase they plume toxic cascades of many different vascular inflammatory free radicals, which attach and expand endothelial and capillary cell basement membrane inflammation. Insulin resistance not only increases blood sugars, but also advanced glycation end products (AGEs), small particle LDL cholesterol, non HDL cholesterol, triglycerides and homocysteine among others. These free radicals also mess with cellular metabolism as they bias fermentation of gluconeogenesis over-glycolysis and the use by mitochondria of fatty acids over pyruvate to produce acetyl CoA. All of these metabolic adjustments that occur from elevated blood sugars increase inflammation through different mechanics resulting in an unstable interstitial space.

Adult diabetes is primarily caused from sloppy behavioral choices involving diet, exercise, and sleep. This means that as we age, we must become more intentional about exercise, fit full sleep and proper diet. Daily routines that highlight eating plant based whole food, regular aerobic and anaerobic exercise, effective sleep hygiene and stress reduction can prevent the blood sugar spiral.

Pre diabetes and adult diabetes represent a worsening continuum of elevated blood sugars. The diabetic spectrum is defined by a blood test known as *hemoglobin A1C*. In truth, anyone over 50 years of age should consider themselves pre diabetic and make preemptive lifestyle choices. In practical terms, the lower the hemoglobin A1C, the less inflammation that is occurring from blood sugar metabolism.

Prediabetes is diagnosed when fasting (no food ingestion for 8 hours or longer) blood sugars fall between 101 and 125 mg /dl *and* hemoglobin A1C is measured between 5.7 and 6.4. Diabetes is diagnosed when the fasting blood sugars are 126 mg/dl or greater and the hemoglobin A C increases to 6.5 or greater. Vascular inflammation caused by elevated blood sugars, and its assortment of co-linked vascular inflammatory free radicals, is a continuum that escalates as hemoglobin A1C increases in the blood. Vascular inflammation can begin as hemoglobin A1C s increases above 5.5, begins to accelerate at 6.5 and then accelerates even faster above 7.0. This makes the inflammatory curve associated with hemoglobin A1C appear logarithmic (see appendix, graph 2). The higher the hemoglobin A1C, the faster inflammation occurs within interstitial spaces. This inflammation involves endothelial and capillary cell basement membranes in all interstitial spaces and end organs throughout the vascular tree.

Diabetes, like smoking tobacco, produces a many splendored cast of free inflammatory free radicals, that increase as hemoglobin A1C levels increase. Adult diabetes has a devastating effect on liver and fat cells. Not only do fat cells grow and multiply in abdominal pannus to influence metabolic momentum, but liver cells will transition to become more like fat cells (*fatty metamorphosis*). When this occurs, liver cells forfeit swaths of their manufacturing and distribution duties. It also causes the liver to produce more proinflammatory free radicals. Many of these will circulate in the bloodstream, penetrate into interstitial spaces, and further expand inflammation.

As blood sugars and hemoglobin A1C increase, liver derived *HSCRP* (highly sensitive c reactive protein) becomes a blood marker of *inflammatory expansion and momentum.* The higher the number, the more interstitial spaces are seething with inflammation. Within the context of diabetes, elevated HSCRP is often linked to the transition of *fatty liver and the metabolic syndrome.* This proinflammatory maladjustment cascades to negatively affect what the liver can manufacture and distribute, which then cascades to adversely affect other end organs. The metabolic syndrome is simply a full blown adult diabetes metabolic mosaic, where all potential vascular inflammatory free radicals are activated and abundant. With metabolic syndrome, not only are blood sugars elevated, but the *basal metabolic index* (BMI) often exceeds 35, blood pressures have risen to 140/90 or greater, and LDL cholesterol, non HDL cholesterol and triglycerides are all elevated in the blood.

Diabetes, or the more virulent metabolic syndrome, is not just about elevated blood sugars but the cascades of different vascular free radicals that impinge endothelial basement membranes while disrupting intracellular metabolism. By fundamentally altering the intercellular mechanics of glucose, pyruvate and fatty acid metabolism, diabetes disrupts feedback loops crosstalk within all cells including endothelial and capillary cells. Intracellular fermentation favors gluconeogenesis over glycolysis and often fatty acids over pyruvate in mitochondrial combustion. This disruption is significant in capillary cells as 90% of their total energy output comes from fermentation.

On outer membranes surfaces, diabetes accentuates inflammation through the genesis of abundant vascular inflammatory free radicals. With AGEs, LDL cholesterol, homocysteine, triglycerides, non HDL cholesterol serving as free radical fuel, they attach to basement membrane surfaces, silence receptors, and plume immune arsenal towards them. In this sense of working in and outside of an endothelial and capillary cell, diabetes becomes a pluripotent proinflammatory disease, a paralyzer to endothelial and capillary cell function.

Diabetes tags onto proinflammatory aging biases that trigger an even faster pace of proinflammatory decline. As people age, there are built- in tendencies to sit, snack, drink alcohol, worry, nap during the day and sleep poorly at night. When coupled with diabetes, all these proinflammatory behaviors increase the speed of inflammatory assault by at least two fold (see index graph one).

As diabetes dismembers endothelial and capillary cell outer membranes and infrastructure, is facilitates the semblance of chronic inflammation within the interstitial space. As such, diabetes supports a robust portfolio of different disease venues in different end organs. In some thrombosis, clots and hypoxic-ischemia may cause the greatest end organ decimation. In others, it could be an infectious disease, cancer of autoimmune complex disorder. Thus diabetes will increase risk for all disease venues from heart attack and strokes, to blindness, sepsis, different cancers and autoimmune disorders. Diabetes is not just a metabolic or vascular disease.

What are the mechanics of free radical attachment to membrane surfaces? Attached small particle LDL cholesterol, not only diminishes basement membrane responsiveness to purposed signals, but they also induce the activation of *RAGE receptors*. Activated RAGE increases endothelial and capillary cell outer membrane permeability of immune arsenal trafficking. When LDL cholesterol continues to activate RAGE, outer membrane protein kinase switches remain on as cAMP is reduced. Outer membrane permeability to immune arsenal persistently increases thereby blocking the capillary cell pivot and swing dance. Persistent RAGE activation which blocks the capillary cell dance and places the interstitial space into a chronic inflammatory cage.

In summary, the diverse array of vascular inflammatory free radicals from adult diabetes pummels endothelial and capillary cell outer membranes and infrastructure to expand inflammation while also blocking endothelial and capillary cell feedback loops that are critical to interstitial space and end organ homeostasis. Instead, these blocked feedback loops are replaced by those derived from rebel immune arsenal thereby creating a different precedent within the interstitial space favoring a chronic inflammatory agenda. With the spewing of free radicals into interstitial spaces, as a result of adult diabetes, chronic inflammation unleashes a perfect storm or proinflammatory momentum. With proinflammatory disruption to endothelia coming at so many different levels, adult diabetes, like tobacco smoke, becomes an ultimate age accelerator. It will cascade proinflammatory momentum in every end organ.

Leptin and Ghrelin

In the obese, or those with adult diabetes or metabolic syndrome the aggregates of inflammatory free radicals and metabolic aberrations cause a net decrease in the circulating hormone *leptin* while increasing its counterpart *ghrelin*. The abnormal ratio feeds back to the brain's satiety center to increase hunger even though not the case. Instead of feeling satisfied, there is desire to eat more even when not required. This becomes particularly true with sugar. In the obese or those with adult diabetes, one cookie or donut can easily escalate to a box of cookies or several donuts. Weight gain can be dramatic leading to a dangerous metabolic hyperbola. As the desire for sugar escalates, vegetables are eschewed in favor of white flour, salt, sugar and trans-fats. This nutritional estrangement cascades a rigorous proinflammatory momentum which often goes unrecognized by the sugar addict. As the leptin/ghrelin ration decreases, the malignant diet of sugar and processed carbs disrupts the intestinal microbiome to propagate substantial leaky gut. The sugar binging eventually increase abdominal adipose and cause liver cell fatty metamorphosis. When liver cells no longer behave as liver cells, the immune compromise caused by poor eating habits is well under way.

Within the interstitial spaces of most end organs, the highly processed-sugary diet, and the abnormal leptin-ghrelin ratio it creates, not only increases free radical impingement on basement membranes to activate RAGE receptors, but also induces activation and migration of IL-6 (or *interleukin 6),* and *tumor necrosis factor* (also known as TNF-alpha, or *cachexin)*. Both are potent proinflammatory mediators that propagate inflammatory expansion. When unopposed they will propagate more immune arsenal into the interstitial space, which eventually become hostile towards capillary cell feedback loop intent. As the capillary cell outer membranes become hijacked by hostile feedback loops from rebel immune arsenal, interstitial space disease venues become inevitable outcomes.

Particulates, Gases and Toxins

Chronic inflammation in any end organ's interstitial space can manifest as a result of exposures intentional or otherwise, to inhaled, injected, absorbed, or digested toxins, gases or particulates. Initial exposures, particularly if in small amounts, may not be perceived to cause harm. However, if there are repeated exposure over time, they can generate enough inflammatory free radical fuel to turn the interstitial space over to chronic inflammation.

The list of potentially harmful toxins, gases and inhaled particulates is growing exponentially, particularly as advances in textile manufacturing has created a variety of different plastics, chemicals, fertilizers, and food preservatives.

When these foreign molecules enter the bloodstream, they can generate inflammation within an end organ's interstitial space by:

- Acting as free radicals and attaching to outer membrane surfaces.
- Penetrate into intracellular infrastructure, attach and block feedback loop mechanics.
- Impair outer membrane permeability by affecting transmembrane pressure gradients, pore dynamics as well as active and passive transport mechanics.
- Block feedback loops signals between outer membranes and mitochondria.
- Produce direct free radical damage to nuclear DNA.

Toxins and particulates, and to some extent toxic gases, exert most of their interstitial space proinflammatory effects as free radicals. They penetrate and attach to endothelial and capillary cell basement membrane surfaces, or perhaps outer membranes of the end organ, to silence or disrupt expression of the affected membrane receptor, and plume an immune arsenal response towards them. The persistence of a given exposure usually determines its risk. The attached culprit will cause default to the capillary cell dance and initiate a chain reaction of proinflammatory intent which eventually causes the interstitial space to turn and favor chronic inflammatory feedback loops. The interstitial space gets hijacked as capillary cells zombie, and mesenchymal and end organ cells capitulate to the new interstitial space order.

As the proinflammatory pieces come together, end organ disease venues emerge, and the capillary cell pseudocapillarizes outer membrane receptors and sharply reduced mitochondrial volumes. All this comes together as rebel and alternative feedback loops channels, synchronized to disease venues, are working overtime within the interstitial space.

When toxin, noxious gas or particulate exposures are coupled with other metabolic vascular inflammatory free radicals (such as AGES, LDL cholesterol, lipo(a)), chronic inflammatory interstitial space momentum accelerates. The message is clear. Any prolonged toxic exposure will stack the table against us. If occurring in the setting of adult diabetes, or a dyslipidemia, proinflammatory momentum will be even faster. The venerable capillary cell dance will be one of the first victims. In the grand scheme, the interstitial space falls to darker influences whose disease outcomes narrow the gap between life and death.

Stress and Sleep Deprivation

Too much stress or not enough sleep have the same impact on chronic inflammatory interstitial space momentum. They will cause maladjustment of adrenal and other hormones that chain react increases in fluid retention, blood pressures, insulin resistance and increases in ghrelin leading to binge overeating and weight gain. There is also evidence that excessive stress and sleep deprivation increases pain and fatigue thereby increasing risk for opioid, antianxiety and sleeping pill addictions.

In other words, stress and sleep disorders push the envelope leading to a tsunami of vascular inflammatory free radical seeds into interstitial spaces. Similar to what can occur with addictions, any combination of prolonged stress and sleep deprivation will chain react increases in metabolic and other free radicals that perpetuates even more stress and sleep deprivation. These inevitably increases fatigue and pain which then chain reacts other proinflammatory behaviors, such as overeating, tobacco or alcohol abuse and often prescription addictions to sleeping pills, anti-anxiety and pain killers. Exercise is postponed indefinitely to favor comfort food. The add-on behaviors self- perpetuate more stress and sleep deprivation as weight increases and obesity becomes morbid. As weight is gained, the sleep deprivation becomes more sinister as *obstructive sleep apnea* fuels further insomnia and disrupted sleep while increasing risks for strokes, atrial fibrillation and heart attacks.

We fail at managing stress or sleep deprivation because we prefer to *react* rather than *confront*. Rather than making intentional adjustments to preempt stress or sleep deprivation, we grind along with the same stressful job, difficult marriage or deeply troubled finances. Instead of change we cope by a few more beers, an extra helping of potatoes or some late night TV. None of these choices help long term.

Just like any other vascular inflammatory free radical, given enough time, stress and sleep deprivation will contribute to chronic inflammatory disease venues, acting as co –contributors within the realm of the anti-organ. It is not uncommon for stress to enable cancer to suddenly show itself or for an autoimmune disease, such as rheumatoid arthritis or lupus, to suddenly become virulent. Stress is underestimated as an inducer of serious interstitial space disease.

To better manage stress, we must become more intentional about eliminating its root cause. A job may need changing, debt may need restructuring, or a relationship a new makeover. A property may need to be sold and a living environment simplified. It also means taking stock of behaviors that have crept into our daily lives and used as coping mechanisms. The morning donut, the afternoon nap, the nightly scotch habit or skipping the afternoon walk will need to be readdressed.

So stress breeds sleep deprivation, and sleep disturbances troll more stress. The cycle produces a reactionary momentum that makes us feel we have little control of life's outcomes. We feel trapped. That's when we turn to sugar, alcohol and drugs for support. Advanced age throws another wrinkle into the equation as it biases lighter sleep, more bathroom interruptions and more anxiety-worry.

Stress and sleep deprivation will cause binge overeating and weight gain, which then increases metabolic free radicals, insulin resistance, blood pressure and sleep apnea. Obstructive sleep apnea (OSA) is a dangerous sleep disturbance that further aggravates sleep deprivation. In those predisposed, OSA will occur as we fall into a deeper level of sleep. The movement of air through the back of our throat gets blocked, causing oxygen levels to decrease in our blood to dangerous levels. As we become hypoxic, we are awakened suddenly by an arousal, which is a reflex signal generated by the brain to start breathing. By awakening, breathing is restored by at the expense of efficient sleep architecture.

Over the course of an evening, total sleep minutes, particularly in the more fit full deep sleep, are substantially decreased. We wake up fatigued, and with brain fog, while increasing risk for sleep induced mini strokes, heart attacks, or abnormal heart rhythms, such as atrial fibrillation. OSA can be treated with a positive pressure face mask titrated to an individual's given need. The best way to prevent OA and its dangerous proinflammatory cascades is to stay fit and keep weight as close to ideal as possible.

Most of us do not possess enough foresight to anticipate how certain activities can cascade the stress mosaic. Becoming more aware of how certain behaviors can affect proinflammatory cascades will go a long way in preempting stress chain reactions. Getting to root causes of why we do things may require deeper introspection. When in doubt, circle back to things that matter most and make adjustments to resolve any family or marital conflict. Letting interpersonal conflicts to fester usually does not play out well and attempts at resolving issues before they escalate are best for improving stress and sleep deprivation. It pays to learn how to identify and problem solve amongst family members and colleagues early and often.

CHAPTER 8

THE PARABLE OF THE WIND AND SEA

There is a place where land, air and sea comingle seamlessly, yet no two days are alike. Each day the sun rises and sets in a different trajectory setting in motion a daily change in light exposure and ambient air temperature. Together with prevailing breezes brings about change in atmospheric conditions which then determines the weather. The different combinations of light, heat and wind over water and land mosaic different cloud formations and propensity for moisture to fall from the sky.

On most days, as the sun rises, it heats up the land surface. As it does, winds develop and push the warm air from the land mass to over the sea, where heat and moisture forms clouds. Predictable rains develop in the late afternoon, and then break up as the sun sets and the temperature cools.

Occasionally this pattern changes, sometimes dramatically. When the sun's trajectory forms the longest long arc of daylight, it produces more light and heat than other days. On this day, the land surface heats to very warm temperatures, and the winds become gusty. The heated air moves from land to sea briskly causing high plumes of clouds stretching tens of thousands of feet into the sky. As the clouds thicken and become darker, lightning flashes can be seen and thunder heard. On this afternoon the sky darkens, and except for the distant thunder, things become quiet, as if dusk coming early.

Suddenly there is an explosive wind gust, soon followed by a continuous very forceful wind. The wind uproots everything stationary to make everything move in the opposite direction. The wind is followed by horizontal rain in sheets and massive water surges. The force of the wind and water surge pushes on everything where nothing stays where it was. Everything moves, topples or tips.

Then suddenly there is complete quiet. The sun peeps out before once again finding cover. Then, as the sky darkened once again, the winds would gust, the rain pelts, and the water surges even more than previously. After some time, it all subsides, this time for good.

Over weeks, life reemerges in the land, air and sea. Predictable patterns that are set by the sun's arc in the sky, and the subsequent light and temperature it generates, reset daily to produce a symbiosis of wind, cloud cover and rain. On these days, conditions would not favor thunder, lightning or strong winds.

Can you interpret the parable? The land mass is the end organ, the sea is the capillary cell and the sun represents our consciousness. The atmospheric conditions, that include ambient air temperature, winds and cloud formation is the interstitial space. In the parable, the sun's arc and the light, heat and winds it produced parallel lifestyle choices and the vascular inflammatory free radical fuel that subsequently migrates into interstitial spaces. The wind gusts and the formation of storm clouds represent outcomes to proinflammatory lifestyle decisions.

As the hurricane matures, it brings together atmospheric conditions that include warm humid air, clouds, lightning and thunder to form a very large storm. This is similar to how chronic inflammation brings together a coalition of rebel immune arsenal (white blood cells, platelets, immunoglobulins) fueled by vascular inflammatory free radicals to cause a powerful interstitial space storm. The unleashing of rain, wind and storm surge coincides with how chronic inflammation can storm surge decimation to the interstitial space.

Eventually the storm dissipates and there is recovery. Similarly, if proinflammatory lifestyle choices are eliminated, the capillary cell dance is restored and the interstitial space may once again become whole.

Life returns to the end organ, just as life on land finds a new footing after the hurricane. Just as atmospheric conditions key the return of an optimal relationship between sun, sea and land, keeping the interstitial space free or vascular inflammatory free radicals enables the capillary cell to reestablish feedback loop intimacy with its end organ and interstitial space allies.

CHAPTER 9

THE BAD AND UGLY OF CHRONIC INFLAMMATION

Regardless of what vascular inflammatory free radicals are involved, their persistence within any interstitial space will eventually cause reckless trafficking of immune arsenal towards them. If free radicals are not eliminated or allowed to smolder within interstitial spaces, reckless immune arsenal trafficking becomes a forgone conclusion. The breakdown of the capillary cell dance is soon followed by a host of proinflammatory chain reactions culminating in interstitial space disease venues.

And this proinflammatory momentum is not isolated to a single interstitial space but occurs everywhere to involve multiple end organs. Chronic interstitial space inflammation causes all end organs to disintegrate and age at a similar pace but with potentially different disease venues.

The monkey wrench of chronic inflammatory control of the interstitial space is how it uses wayward immune arsenal to evolve an alternative feedback loop communication system which supersedes the increasingly crippled capillary cell network. The feedback loops perpetuate chronic inflammatory intent while propping up its defenses at the expense of the end organ. Capillary cell immune arsenal choreography into interstitial spaces is replaced by a different choreography suitable to anti-organ disease venues.

When capillary cells cave, the interstitial space becomes a dark and foreboding place to the interests of the end organ. It is in this dark cavern that anti-organ disease venues proliferate. It is at this "end stage" of chronic inflammation that we base current Osler driven disease treatment models.

Sepsis-Bacterial control of Interstitial Space Free Fall

When bacteria or other infectious agents are enabled by the chronic inflammatory apparatus to hide, or multiply in stealth within the interstitial space, they become a reservoir for sepsis. Sepsis is defined as the spread of an infectious agent into the blood stream that is usually accompanied by hypotension and fever. For example, as bacteria multiply within the interstitial space, they can not only overwhelm the interstitial space where they are nesting, but can leak into the blood stream to invade other interstitial spaces and end organs. When bacteria can move freely from an interstitial space to and from the blood stream, there effects can be life threatening. Before the antibiotic era, sepsis was often diagnosed late and carried a mortality exceeding 90%. Within the last 25 years, sepsis is diagnosed much earlier in the clinical course and carries an expected mortality of about 15% in those that are resuscitated from shock.

Sepsis becomes dangerous when bacteria secrete substances (*endotoxins*) that cause fever, hypotension, hypoxia and interstitial edema fluid, also known as *third spacing*. In combination with a rapidly progressive bacterial population, the interstitial space of the involved end organ if often flogged in chaos with combinations of proliferating white blood cells, immunoglobulins platelets and clotting factors, all of which in combination with endotoxin, make the space even more deadly. In this setting, antibiotics have been a game changer in stemming the massive bacterial overgrowth.

Sepsis causes much of its disruption through the release of endotoxin. Endotoxin has a profound impact on endothelial cell permeability. Eventually sequencing choreography of immune arsenal gives way en bloc mobilization into the interstitial space, accompanied by large volumes of albumin, clotting factors, complement and edema fluid. If sepsis is not managed aggressively enough with antibiotics, the affected end organ can fail, the infection can smolder, become chronic or recurrent, or scar tissue can form from nearby mesenchymal cells. An interstitial space that chronically harbors bacteria becomes a setup for cancer growth, autoimmune complex disease or thrombosis leading to hypoxic -ischemic events. Any or all of these will compromise the end organ. The sepsis endotoxin model occurs from bacterial infections, but sepsis can also occur from viruses, parasites, fungi or combinations of different infectious agents.

Sepsis is more likely to occur when chronic inflammation has established a foothold within the interstitial space. When chronic inflammation has succeeded in causing the production of fibrous scar tissue, bacteria or other infectious agents are more likely to find hiding places within the scar tissue to grow and multiply. Scarring also makes it harder to immune arsenal to penetrate and recognize and invader. Interstitial space scarring, coupled with bacterial or viral seeding, create a perfect combination that mutually supports each other's development. These relationships are common seen with infections of the bladder, gums, lung and kidney but can involve any end organ. Eventually cancer growth can also take advantage of this symbiosis.

Implied in sepsis vulnerability is the vascular inflammatory free radical fuel that serves as the foundation to chronic inflammatory interstitial space and basement membrane impingement. Sepsis takes another leg up with advanced age, due to aggregate combinations of end organ interstitial space scarring, the bias towards endothelial cell outer membrane receptor silencing, and the crosslinked nuclear DNA which has silenced so much protein synthesis replacement.

The most commonly studied endotoxin is *LPS* (lipopolysaccharides). LPS can forge sepsis through a massive induction of non -sequenced capillary cell permeability. LPS both distracts and makes it harder for endothelia to identify and then induce an immune arsenal response that will focus on a bacterial kill shot. Instead, the inflammatory response gets misdirected and often needs antimicrobial back-up to contain and eliminate the offending organism. LPS causes a dramatic interstitial space expansion of neutrophils and inflammatory cytokines such as IL-6, CRP *(C-reactive protein)*, as well as *thromboxane A-2* and *thrombin*. These inflammatory mediators surge into the interstitial space, and cause secondary increases in edema fluid and pro-clotting biases, while also constricting the lumens of downstream arterioles to *decrease* blood flow to an already oxygen compromised end organ.

One thing becomes clear from this discussion. As anti-organ disease venues, including bacteria and other infectious agents, populate the interstitial space, they make the space vulnerable to additional disease venues. Chronic infectious influences within the interstitial space increase risk for scarring, thrombosis, cancer or autoimmune disease, while each of these also increases the risk for infections. The late consequences of chronic inflammation and the disabled immune trafficking they cause, make it more likely that a variety of different disease venues will occur within a given end organ's interstitial space, before the end organ tanks and calls it quits.

Thrombosis: The Gateway to End Organ Death

Thrombosis is the culmination of a clot and constitutes different combinations of inflammatory debris, clotting factors, and platelets. In the setting of chronic inflammation, biases are set in motion within interstitial spaces which accentuate clotting. Thrombosis exemplifies the capillary cell double whammy conundrum. As obstructive plaque and basement membrane thickening increase in larger blood vessels downstream, they not only increase risks for thrombosis and a complete blood cut off but also limit the upstream capillary cell from responding appropriately to end organ on demand oxygen signals.

In most cases, the clinical drama leading up to a large vessel thrombosis is one of slow torture, as upstream capillaries struggle to improve oxygen delivery to a chronically compromised end organ. As blood flows and oxygen levels diminish to the end organ, the interstitial space not only suffers from the consequences of hypoxia, but the end organ typically atrophies as amyloid and scar tissue are secreted from mensenchymal cells. This is classically found in brain shrinkage in dementia, as blood flow and oxygen delivery evaporate.

Pro-clotting tendencies will be biased to occur with any disease venues within the interstitial space. An interstitial space riddled with cancer growth or infection will be ripe for clotting venues. The genesis of pro clotting biases has several different origins, from the cancer and bacterial cells themselves, inducing a pro -clotting prodrome, to the chronically inflamed and thickened basement membrane surfaces, which attract clotting factors and platelets. As expected, this proinflammatoriy momentum does little to restore the capillary cell dance or reset mitochondrial combustion to nitric oxide.

Pro clotting biases escalate within interstitial spaces on the basis of blocked capillary cell choreography. Clotting factors and platelets not only randomly descend into the interstitial space, but are activated by rogue signals within the interstitial space to initiate thrombosis. Vascular inflammatory free radicals (such as small particle LDL cholesterol among others) attach to basement membranes and expand rebel white blood cell and cytokine (such as IL-6) directives, which further fuel pro clotting biases. Regardless of where the clot(s) occur, when instigated by chronic inflammation, there is oxygen cutoff and sudden end organ compromise from hypoxia.

Thrombosis of several smaller arterial vessels, can be just as damaging to the end organs as one larger vessel occlusion. The occlusions of smaller vessels can cause a stuttering of end organ declines. The benchmark for this type of occlusion is commonly seen on brain imaging where there are extensive ischemic white matter changes that are associated with progressive memory loss. These changes are often interpreted as normal for age but are anything but normal as it underpins the beginnings of dementia.

Thrombosis and hypoxic ischemic events involving end organs are late outcomes to chronic interstitial space inflammation and are more likely to occur when the chronic inflammatory anti-organ has partitioned the interstitial space off with its own communication system and other disease venues. Since most end organs utilize oxygen to combust energy to perform their functions, with its sudden cut-off a direct assault to their viability. While end organs suffer from lack of oxygen, several disease venues thrive. Such is the case with fibrous scarring, anaerobic bacteria or fermenting cancer cells.

Cancer Cells: From Innocent Bystanders to Interstitial Space Pariah

At any given moment in time our body may harbor hundreds if not thousands of aberrant cancer like cells. When interstitial space sanitation is clicking, implying a vigorous capillary cell dance, cancer cells are quickly id'd and disposed of through normal immune mechanics. This is because the surveillance and feedback loop signaling system within the interstitial space is well versed in their removal. Once id'd, monocytes or mesenchymal cells will remove the cell by engulfing it (phagocytosis). Once engulfed, it is auto digested into basic molecules and recycled.

When the immune system has gone awry on the basis of cracks generated from chronic interstitial space inflammation, cancer cells are not adequately identified and removed. This occurs from the usual buildup of culprits that prevalent in chronic inflammation. The presence of abundant vascular inflammatory free radical fuel, coupled with an increasingly rogue and lackluster interstitial space immune arsenal, and a blocked capillary cell dance and the proinflammatory pieces are in place for a missed choreography. Without proper ID, cancer cells are allowed to escape into interstitial space caverns and go unnoticed. It does not take long for the cell to take advantage of interstitial space dynamics to begin growth. Depending on the context, cancer cells may grow in what would be considered a harsh environment for somatic cells. Among others things, cancer cells can utilize fermentation processes (glycolysis-no oxygen) to support its growth.

After reaching a certain *critical mass*, the cancer entity subspecializes its mass and begins to implement its own defense and surveillance systems, employing rebel immune arsenal and mesenchymal cells in the process. When this proinflammatory interstitial space hyperbola comes to fruition, it's not just cancer growth that occurs, but all its weaponry as well. This includes ample development of fibrous scar tissue, various infectious vulnerabilities, and pro clotting dynamics.

Different cancers grow at different rates depending on well they can nest within the interstitial space and how unresponsive their nucleus has become to blocking replication signals. Rate of growth, or cell division is often based on how primitive their DNA is. Cancer cells whose DNA is more identical to that of the end organ from which they came from generally will grow and multiply more slowly compared to cells whose DNA bears little resemblance. Even so, well differentiated cancers can grow quickly if proinflammatory conditions within the interstitial space favor their growth. This would occur in situations where there is abundant vascular inflammatory free radical fuel within the interstitial space and the capillary cell feedback loops system has been severely crippled. Such would be the case in those with diabetes, cigarette smokers, alcoholics or drug abusers.

As cancer growth matures within interstitial spaces, it becomes its own entity and competes directly with the end organ for oxygen and energy substrate. It establishes its own *symbiosis, meaning its own boundaries and support system*. Part of that symbiosis is to further advance the agendas of chronic inflammation. Together cancer and the anti-organ combine utilities within the interstitial space by comingling their feedback loop communication system that involves rebel immune arsenal and converted mesenchymal cells. This enables cancer to coexist and even thrive as additional anti-organ disease venues are propagated within the interstitial space. As these disease venues mature, the already crippled capillary cell becomes a zombied slave to their new owners, cancer and the anti-organ. Their infrastructure has been gutted as mitochondria and outer membrane receptors have decreased. As capillary cell nitric oxide combustion goes on permanent hiatus, cancer and the anti-organ use capillary cell outer membranes to import into the interstitial space whatever it wants from blood plasma to support its growth at the expense of the end organ.

This is how cancer isolates and kills. By controlling interstitial space feedback loops and dismantling the capillary cell, cancer grows, develops its own symbiosis as well as defense and surveillance systems, making it nearly impossible to penetrate utilizing normal immune mechanics. In this respect, cancer meets the criteria of a saprophyte as it takes from the body what it wants, does not contribute anything of substance in return, and increases deterioration of the end organ from which it came from.

What becomes interesting is how cancer parlays immune arsenal to switch sides. It does this through sneaky subversion of wayward immune arsenal entering the interstitial space without having been sequenced or properly choreographed. These mostly white blood cells send cytokine signals that misdirect the immune arsenal response away from the cancer cell and towards a something else. This feedback loop momentum builds on itself through chain reactions and supported by interstitial space free radical fuel. Over time, immune arsenal gets diverted away from cancer cells to become increasingly hostile towards the capillary and end organ cell outer membranes. As cancer grows its mass its can shed cells without sacrificing its defenses for purposes of metastatic spread.

Like other disease venues, cancer growth relies on a blocked capillary cell dance and abundant vascular inflammatory free radical fuel. Getting these two attributes within the interstitial space creates enough chronic inflammatory momentum to enable cancer cells opportunity to hide and grow.

Autoimmune Complex Disease: One False Step

Autoimmune disorders are families of diseases that are the result of different mistaken identities to normal cellular proteins. That is, proteins that are "normal" functioning proteins on membrane surfaces are attacked by confused immunoglobulins which mistaken them for being foreign or not belonging to the body. In this sense autoimmune disease is not only a case of mistaken identity but also missed opportunity. Good proteins get sacked without good reason while sinister "foreign" proteins belonging to cancer cells, infectious agents or particulates are left alone. This confusion about what proteins immunoglobulins should attack and leave alone is perpetuated by chronic interstitial space inflammation. It is clear, that as chronic inflammation organizes within interstitial spaces one of its weapons of disruption is to confuse immunoglobulins about what to attach to.

When or how chronic inflammation causes immunoglobulins to go rogue is not clear, but it is enabled by cytokine feedback loops from rebel immune arsenal. As immunoglobulins switch allegiance the proinflammatory momentum within the interstitial space has kicked up a series of false feedback loop signals involving misguided cytokines and white blood cells. Together they chain react dark transition within interstitial spaces that turns the space against the end organ. As cytokines, white blood cells, platelets and complement within interstitial spaces are converted by a darker set of feedback loops, not only does aberrant autoimmune complex disease increase but so do other disease venues that involve fibrous scarring, infections, cancer growth and thrombosis. Thus autoimmune complex disease becomes a disease venue that fosters an increased risk for thrombosis (strokes, heart attacks, deep vein thrombosis –leg clot, pulmonary embolus-lung clot), cancers or infections within interstitial spaces.

Just like with the other anti-organ disease venues, immune complex disease has its roots in abundant vascular inflammatory free radical fuel and a blocked capillary cell dance. As immune arsenal is called into the interstitial space to "chase" the ever present free radicals, the capillary cell dance is blocked and nitric oxide combustion limited. The chronic inflammatory round about then begins. As immune arsenal fails to be sequenced or choreographed, their vagabond presence within interstitial spaces becomes the thorn of cytokine rebellion. Eventually with enough cytokine chain reactions at their disposal, chronic inflammation wrestles feedback loop communication away from the endothelial- capillary cell and its allies. The feedback loop communication signaling switch overhauls the entire interstitial space including immunoglobulins and mesenchymal cells and defines the chronic inflammatory matrix. As capillary cell feedback loops are replaced, protection of the interstitial space and preservation of end organ function diminish.

When an immunoglobulin attaches to a protein on a membrane surface, it forms an *antigen-antibody complex.* This complex becomes recognizable as something to eliminate by monocytes or mesenchymal cells. To further prep the complex for removal, it is prepared by the attachment of *complement or other cytokines,* to chain react eventual engulfment by monocytes or mesenchymal cells. Hence the immunoglobulin attachment to a protein, normal or otherwise, cascades a series of reactions culminating in the dissolution of the protein or cell from its origin.

When this protein is form a normal functioning membrane surface, the effects can be devastating. This mistake actually perpetuates through the mechanics of *immune memory,* where similar or identical membrane proteins are mistakenly and systematically attacked and destroyed. The recurrent inflammatory cascade against normal proteins will disrupt membrane function and disable the affected end organ. The inflammatory momentum that builds from these aberrant chain reaction of mistaken identities disrupts interstitial space homeostasis to such a degree that opportunity increases for other anti-organ disease venues to populate.

The compilation of rogue immune complexes can involve multiple end organs through very similar mechanics. Different autoimmune diseases are known by the different types of autoimmune complexes they generate in different end organs. As might be expected, these adverse autoimmune outcomes are less likely to occur, or more likely to be reversed, if there is a reduction of the vascular inflammatory free radical fuel within interstitial spaces. This reduction reverses proinflammatory momentum, which is triggered by the steady return of the capillary cell dance. As capillaries and endothelia dance, mitochondrial combustion is permitted to switch to nitric oxide, which changes the entire capillary cell equation, including the regeneration of its feedback loop communication system with its interstitial space allies.

An emerging theme, that coincides with the obesity epidemic, is the relationship of autoimmune diseases to *adipokines.* Adipokines are a families of inflammatory cytokines secreted from white fat cells (*WAT-white adipose tissue*) which have influences on immune proteins (immunoglobulins), other cytokines and macrophage- white blood cells. With increased obesity and abdominal fat pannus, these abdominal fat cells (WAT) increase in size and volume. As they do, they take on more metabolic precedent as they exert powerful adipokine feedback loops to the liver and other end organs. As circulating adipokines increase in the blood, they begin to affect circulating immunoglobulins by tweaking their configurations and increasing risk for identity mistakes. Once the immunoglobulin mistake is made on a membrane surface protein, it will cascade more mistakes. Adipokines could initiate this cascade by reconfiguring circulating immunoglobulin morphology enabling them to become more mistake prone.

Once the proinflammatory antigen-antibody complex has been initiated by adipokines or through other mechanics, complement and IL- 1 and 6 attachments further mature the antigen- antibody complex, and is followed by *PAI-1 (plasminogen activator-inhibitor type one)*, TNF (tumor necrosis factor) and VEGF (vascular endothelial growth factor). In aggregate they chain react the maturing of the antigen-antibody complex leading to monocyte, macrophage or mesenchymal cell engulfment.

This unwelcome proinflammatory cascade, particularly as it is affected by adipokines, suggests that sugar, obesity, adult diabetes, the metabolic syndrome induce abdominal fat pannus growth that induces autoimmune mistakes. Once autoimmune catastrophes are well established, with enough vascular inflammatory free radical fuel and a sufficiently blocked capillary cell dance, other disease venues will amply take their place in a chaotic interstitial space. Could it be that the best way to cut autoimmune disease to maintain an optimal lean body mass, exercise regularly and sleep well? I dare say a self- repeating pattern of wellness and disease prevention. This revelation may explain why a vegetable based diet, leaner body mass, elimination of addictions, and regular exercise all contribute to *less autoimmune disease.*

Scar Tissue: As It increases, the End Organ Must Decrease

End organ fibrous scar tissue, occurs most often as an outcome to chronic interstitial space inflammation. It is caused by *converted* mesenchymal cells who begin receiving and responding to feedback loops signals from rebel immune arsenal. It is invariably associated with vascular inflammatory free radical buildup within interstitial spaces, a blocked capillary cell dance and a stuck capillary cell mitochondrial combustion in energy. When mesenchymal cells take orders from cells other than capillary cells or traditional allies, they get confused and will do the wrong thing, such as producing scar tissue. Scar tissue can actually be part of a healing process from trauma, but in the context of chronic inflammation, it can be destructive as it further separates the end organ cells from its capillary nurturers. Scar tissue is usually composed of *layers of collagenous fibers* (fibrous scar) or as *amyloid.* Both types, when incorporated into the interstitial spaces of end organs, are relatively inert, take up space from atrophied end organ cells, and require very little oxygen or energy substrate to maintain. They barrier or partition the disabled capillary cell from the shrinking end organ cells.

You could say that the layering of fibrous scar tissue within interstitial spaces is a form of slow end organ torture, as it makes oxygen and energy substrate delivery to the end organ even more tangled that it would be. Like all disease venues, scarring is fueled by vascular inflammatory free radicals, and takes off when mesenchymal cells turn as the result of an alternative feedback loop signaling system.

One way to describe fibrous scar tissue, or amyloid and its cousin tau, is as a type of *filler* that becomes the cause and effect of atrophied or dying end organ cells. As it layers within the interstitial space the fibrous scar tissue or amyloid, not only deters normal exchanges between capillary and end organ cells, but also create ready- made crevices for bacteria, viruses or cancer cells to hide and grow. Finally, scar tissue becomes a nidus for pro-clotting biases and escalating thrombosis within the interstitial space, as platelets and clotting factors find more reasons to become activated. In contractual terms, fibrous scarring becomes the mother lode for the proliferation of other disease venues.

Within interstitial spaces there can be different types of scar tissue but all are composed of different sizes and shapes of collagen fibrils or amyloid. Once secreted, they machinate within interstitial spaces taking on a spider web type of appearance, with varying density and partitions of its fibrils. The fibril mesh does not require much oxygen or nutrient support as it can function as an inert scaffolding entity. Amyloid precipitation has predilection for brain, heart, liver, skin, and kidney. Like fibrous scar tissue, amyloid deposition within interstitial spaces is linked to an already compromised relationship between end organ cells and capillary providers. Its classic presentation in found with decaying and atrophic brain cells and has been linked to various dementias.

The presence of scar tissue is often first noticed in one end organ; for example, in the brain where it is linked to amyloid deposition, brain atrophy and dementia. In fact, however, either amyloid or fibrous scarring can be found simultaneously, with perhaps less progression, in multiple end organs. This is due to vascular inflammatory free radicals, the blocked capillary cell dance and a stuck mitochondrial combustion in energy having no boundaries within the entire human organisms. Typical vascular inflammatory free radical accumulations from diabetes, tobacco, or alcohol and drug abuse occur in every vascular and interstitial space nook and cranny. As such chronic inflammation within those interstitial spaces will eventually elicit scar tissue elsewhere as their playbook turns mesenchymal cells in their neighborhood.

The determination of whether to secrete fibrous scar or amyloid may become a preference based on end organ function or what inherent genetics may predispose. The point being, that unless vascular inflammatory free radicals are substantially reduced to turn the tide on the capillary cell dance and mitochondrial combustion, chronic inflammation will have a field day within interstitial spaces in collaborating with mesenchymal cells to cause scar progression.

Is there a possibility that interstitial space fibrous scarring and amyloid can be reversed? Preliminary investigation suggests the possibility but the cart must not be placed in front of the horse. Removing amyloid without removing vascular inflammatory free radicals will carry no clinical impact. Rather, with the combination of anti-inflammatory lifestyle choices and judicious use of medicinals and supplements, to treat and prevent disease venues and vitamin and antioxidant deficiencies, the possibility of reversing scar tissue becomes more likely. In this setting, the reversal is connected with a return of the capillary cell dance and swinging of combustion to nitric oxide. As scarring reverses, other disease venues become less likely to appear as well. It also means that the end organ will receive more on demand oxygen and nutrient, thereby rejuvenating its function. Fatigue, pain and aging take a back seat.

This proposed hypothesis has profound implications on not just scarring but every disease venue. Implied in reversing inflammatory momentum is a revolution involving a lot of vascular moving parts and feedback loop signaling chain reactions. It involves interstitial spaces from the largest of arterial vessels to the smallest of capillaries. In short, scar reversal, like any disease venue reversal, requires a rigorous and intentional anti-inflammatory momentum generated by lifestyle to outcome wellness. Central to returned viability is the fully functioning capillary cell dance.

Chronic and Debilitating Fatigue: The Underbelly of the Anti-Organ

No matter which end organ headlines a disease venue, as it deteriorates, fatigue increases. Because fatigue is so common with aging, it generally gets dismissed as age related wearing out. While aging does contribute to fatigue, it is fa less of an issue than that of chronic inflammation.

Fatigue is described as having less capacity or endurance to do what we think we should. In many respects, fatigue becomes self- fulfilling as the less we do, the less we want to do. Before you know it, we sit more because that is all we are capable of doing. The more we sit, the more effort that is required to stand and walk.

The causes of fatigue, on the surface can look complex, as we divvy up different end organ functions and attempt dissection of their failures, failing to recognize one common cause-chronic inflammation. It is further nuanced by consistently poor lifestyle choices that include too much stress, too little exercise, sugar holicism, and lack of sleep. While too much or too little of end organ function contributes to fatigue (such as thyroid disorders), the bigger picture, we cause most of our own fatigue. Further, the proinflammatory momentum that adverse lifestyle choices cause, will "a fait de accompli" end organ dysfunctions, thereby becoming a self- fulfilling prophesy. Fatigue wins when we become to brain fogged by our lifestyle that we lose capacity to identify root causes

When we lose focus on what we are doing to ourselves, or worse, get to the point where we think it no longer matters, fatigue wins in spades. We are, in essence, asking chronic inflammation to take charge of our interstitial spaces. As chronic inflammation matures within interstitial spaces and disease venues within end organs mount, unrelenting fatigue will feed on itself. This means more sitting, fast food, weight gain, less sleep and more stress. Taking medicines to combat outcomes to bad behaviors, only produces a minor blimp in the chronic fatigue progression.

These proinflammatory cascades not only imply lifestyle choices as cause and effect but also suggest that our choices become increasingly reactive and less intentional as fatigue escalates. We become more like a ping pong ball, bouncing from one bad to choice to another. Before we know it we are in the throws of the medical industrial complex with tests, procedures and drugs and no way out. We suffocate from combinations of our girth, prescriptions drugs and endless tests, which in some perverted way, makes up comfortable in feeling taken care of. Unfortunately, short term benefits in treatment an d improved fatigue are usually squandered by additional lifestyle mistakes, which fail to be taken seriously by the medical industrial complex. How much time does the average practitioner spend with patients taking about the mechanics of sleep hygiene, sugar gateways, alcohol addiction, stress mediation or appropriate levels of exercise? As we take our drugs and do out tests to treat our illnesses, we become increasingly dependent on wrong somethings or cascades of wrong somethings. We love putting the cart before the horse. As a result, chronic fatigue *chain reacts* from escalating disease venues that are caused by chronic interstitial space inflammation and involve multiple end organs.

How can we break this cycle that spirals debilitating fatigue? Like a broken record, it comes down to recognizing and reducing the fuel of chronic inflammation. If we can make the connection of lifestyle to chronic inflammatory free radical fuel, the maturing of chronic interstitial space inflammation, disease venues and debilitating fatigue, we can begin the discussion of wellness and healing.

A recurring theme in *Trafficking* as well as in my first two books, *Hazing Aging and Rejuvenation!* is that chronic inflammation breads from the chronic dispersal of vascular inflammatory free radicals that stem from poor lifestyle choices. These free radicals get dumped into interstitial spaces and impinge on endothelial cell basement membranes where they begin the process of neutering well intentioned immune arsenal. As they protagonize incoming immune arsenal, the block the capillary cell dance, and mitochondrial nitric oxide combustion. Eventually mitochondrial volumes self -destruct form their own superoxide exhaust, and outer membranes follow suit as the pseudocapillarize their surfaces. The combination invites the chronic inflammatory matrix to turn up the interstitial space heat and pirate the feedback loop communication signaling network away from the blighted capillary cell. Disease venues escalate, end organ function is marginalized and chronic fatigue bounces.

Reversal of fatigue, requires reversal of disease venues, which requires reversal of chronic inflammation, which requires capillary cells to dance. This requires a sharp reduction in vascular inflammatory free radical fuel, which enables the by now meager capillary cell outer membranes to signal their diminished mitochondria to combust nitric oxide. The swing in combustion begins interstitial space renewal. As capillary mitochondrial combustion swings to nitric oxide, capillaries find their mojo. Interstitial space hygiene and end organ viability soon follow. Fatigue remits.

In outdated disease treatment models, we think of fatigue as a result of an end organ disease venue. If we treat end organ disease, we improve fatigue. For example, if the heart is causing fatigue because it does not contract well, if we improve heart contraction fatigue improves. What we don't do very well, it gets down to the mechanics of why the heart is not pumping well enough. If we don't get there and make those corrections, disease treatments will be short lived and require even more disease treatment in a vicious cycle. You can plug any end organ into this disease treatment model with similar outcomes. Treating dementia with drugs to increase different neurotransmitters known to be deficient in dementia, will work for a while, until the underlying chronic inflammation will make drug supplementing refractory to dementia treatment. The same holds true for drugs that eliminate amyloid or tau buildup. Without addressing root causes of chronic inflammation within the brain, these treatments will be futile.

In contrast to the Osler *disease treatment model*, the *chronic inflammatory model*, infers that fatigue is not just the result of one or even two failed end organs, but rather occurs from inflammatory processes in the interstitial spaces of multiple end organs. To make fatigue go away, holistic lifestyle choices must be front burnered, chronic inflammation directly assaulted, *and then* coupled with interspersed disease treatment. This puts the horse back in front of the cart where it belongs. Fatigue melts as energy escapes in ways we have not felt in decades. The sooner the transition, the better.

Chronic Pain

Treating chronic pain in disease treatment models has been a colossal failure. The addicting and pain tolerance affects, from narcotic pain relievers, has caused a serous opioid epidemic, with millions of lives lost from both prescription and street drug abuses. In addition, narcotics can gateway other addictions that involve sleeping pills, anti-anxiety treatments, sugar and alcohol. Increasing tolerance to their pain relieving effects, biases further escalation in dose, and the serious psychological effects that follow. The addicting co-combinations of different drugs escalate rather than reduce chronic interstitial space inflammation. Thus pain management, no matter how altruistic, causes more chronic inflammatory harm than the pain relief they treat.

Without treating chronic inflammation any pain management will eventually fail. Substituting opioids for acetaminophen, or nonsteroidal anti-inflammatories (NSAIDS) like ibuprofen, only exchange one set of serious side effects for another, without addressing chronic inflammation. The debate will continue to rage as to whether pain drugs cause more deaths and disability than the purported disease symptoms they are treating. For purposes of discussion it must be pointed out that in the management of acute pain, all pain armamentarium should be employed. It is in chronic pain management where all of the choices produce black holes.

Like chronic fatigue, its sister chronic pain, is associated with the maturing of chronic interstitial space inflammation and the development of end organ disease venues. Also like chronic fatigue, the finger of chronic pain is often pointed at one effected end organ, such as the lumbar spine (lumbago), knee or hip arthritis, a cancer diagnosis, or an autoimmune complex disease rather than the broad scope of chronic inflammation and how it impacts all end organs. While we desire to blame pain on a bone on bone knees or hip, we prefer to ignore the weight gain, diabetes, and tobacco abuse that produced enough chronic inflammation to make the pain intolerable. The fact is that lifestyle adjustments in diet, exercise and weight loss will reverse the majority of bone on bone joint pains without surgery. On the other hand, having joint replacement surgery without addressing lifestyle will have short lived results.

It is clear that chronic pain treatment needs a makeover. In the wellness era, pain is treated dually by reducing inflammation first with exercise, diet and sleep improvements and then supplementing this management with lesser invasive pain treatment. This might take the form of topically applied creams or gels, different joint wraps, stretching and changing exercise routines to favor less joint trauma.

This type of pain management is more difficult but better as it places the onus for improvement on the motivation of the patient. In other words, the patient becomes intentional about the process rather than reactive, which becomes the first pillar of wellness. Making the patient responsible to chronic pain management, rather than just popping an addictive pill and forgetting about it, becomes the new era of pain management. This approach does not produce a day and night difference in pain but over time will cause improvement. This truly does require a cultural shift in our on demand desire for treatment of anything that bothers us.

Are we ready for a cultural shift in chronic pain management? Pain management becomes just the tip of the iceberg, as doing so will require more direct attention to chronic inflammation which will then change the dynamics of how disease gets managed. Minimizing vascular inflammatory free radicals becomes the gateway to preventing and treating all disease venues as well as the foundational floor plan for chronic pain management.

Advanced Age and the 2-3X Effect on Chronic inflammation

Advanced age is a relative term. While we think of advanced age as those over 65 years of age there are those who have advanced age at 45, while there are others that don't have evidence for advanced age at 85 or even 90. If we look at averages however, advanced age fits the definition for most people in western culture as being over 75 years of age with the common denominator being the piling up of chronic illnesses.

The implication about advanced age is that it involves increasing genetic damage, silencing of protein synthesis, and increased vulnerability, because of these silenced proteins, to the effects of chronic inflammation. Cells simply lose quality assurance as they age. Certain things just don't get done which opens the door for inflammatory risks.

Because capillary cells stem and pace interstitial space hygiene and end organ function, their loss of outer membrane protein receptors and mitochondria that come about from aging is particularly risky. The bias for capillary cell DNA degradation has its origins with vascular inflammatory free radicals. As capillaries and their mitochondria spend more time combusting energy to combat the free radical pestilence, they spend less time in nitric oxide combustion and more time making superoxide exhaust. Less nitric oxide means less repair and replacement. More superoxide means more membrane and nuclear DNA damage. The double whammy accelerates chronic inflammatory intent.

With fewer outer membrane receptors and a far less capable mitochondrial network, capillary cells cannot generate a strong feedback loop communication link with their interstitial space partners (mesenchymal cells and end organs). As these communication links whither and are replaced by a more hostile feedback loop system from emerging rebel immune arsenal, the interstitial space, immune arsenal and mesenchymal cells fall in line and the interstitial space chronic inflammatory coupe occurs seamlessly. As the interstitial space transitions disease venues populate. The end organ is forced to withdraw function as their mitochondria become increasingly stuck in nitric oxide combustion and the production of toxic hydroxynitrile (cousin of cyanide) free radical exhaust.

Therefore, the aging effect in capillary cells, is about how the accumulation of DNA damage over time nuances further exploitation by chronic inflammation. The interstitial space anti-organ will use all of the discrepancy caused from ineffective capillary cell DNA coding to its benefit. Thus with advanced age any sustained uptick in vascular inflammatory free radical impingement within interstitial spaces of end organs will unleash a much more potent effect on basement membranes and induce a faster pace towards disease venues.

Aging has another troublesome wrinkle. In addition to what I have mentioned, aging is also linked to reductions in antioxidant levels that neutralize free radicals. These reductions cause a greater lingering of free radicals in most spaces including those that could attach to infrastructure or nuclear DNA. Antioxidant reductions serve as further fuel to free radical toxicity.

With aging, antioxidants decrease from combinations of reduced intestinal tract *absorption*, ineffective *production or overutilization*. Regardless of what causes their reduction they become less effective in free radical neutralization. Age related antioxidant deficiency is one more mechanism that favors anti-organ momentum.

To tackle proinflammatory biases connected with advanced age, disciplined and intentional lifestyle intervention is essential. Even occasional cheating will have its price. The point is simple. Age requires a reset of anti-inflammatory *prognostication* as proinflammatory influences stack against it.

CHAPTER 10

THE MAKING OF INTERSTITIAL SPACE SANITATION: HOW CAPILLARY—ENDOTHELIAL CELL ANATOMY ARCHIVES IMMUNE ARSENAL TRAFFICKING

The First Layer of Capillary Cell Outer Membrane Quality Assurance: the Glycocalyx

The front line of capillary cell trafficking of immune arsenal into interstitial spaces is the first of three outer membrane surfaces known as the luminal *glycocalyx* (see the corresponding figure below). The glycocalyx is an flexible luminal membrane composed of dense fiber-like mesh that fluxes its configuration and thickness to expose different receptor attachments. Fluxing is based on cross current momentum based on signaling messages from the interstitial space (opposite or *abluminal side* of the endothelial and capillary cell) and end organ. A well- kept capillary cell has a thick and well -defined glycocalyx. Its thickness helps mosaic different immune arsenal attachments and barrier the capillary cell continuous outer membrane from blood plasma constituents. As such, the glycocalyx further wrinkles capillary cell choreography to assist in the mosaic of *staging* of an immune arsenal response to interstitial space inflammatory breach.

As might be expected, in some end organs, the capillary cell glycocalyx is thick and well defined, whereas in others (liver sinusoid) it is less so. Generally, as capillary cells become increasingly dysfunctional from chronic interstitial space inflammation, their glycocalcyx thins and loses ability to mosaic animmune arsenal response.

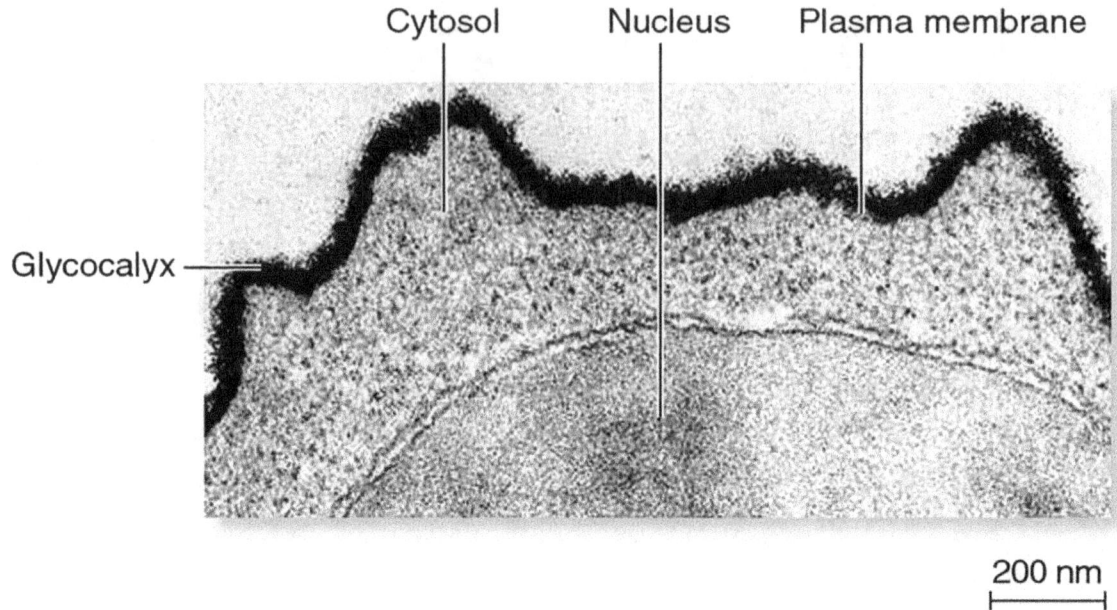

The glycocalyx affects capillary cell trafficking in at least three different ways:

- It provides *feedback loop momentum* to the capillary cell pivot and swing dance by bringing synergies to outer membrane messaging to further promote successful staging of an inflammatory response. Doing so promotes a more robust response to capillary cell intended purpose while supporting its feedback loop communication system with the interstitial space and its allies. The glycocalcyx therefore increases the likelihood of a successful response to inflammatory breach removal, which then enables the capillary endothelia to pivot permeability and swing combustion.
- Helps to nuance fluid and electrolyte movement into and out of the capillary cell thereby producing a built in quality assurance to optimal capillary cell cytoplasmic homeostasis. In this sense the glycocalyx acts as a first-line fluid and electrolyte membrane filter.
- Further nuances the pace of immune arsenal sequencing into the interstitial space through combinations of mesh flexing and bending mechanics, different membrane receptor exposures and modifying its electromechanical gradient.

The feedback loop relationship the glycocalyx has with capillary cell mitochondrial combustion is nuanced in different ways. Mitochondrial energy or nitric oxide combustion can be biased in one direction or the other by how dynamic the glycocalyx responds to luminal *shear stress, interstitial space inflammatory signals*, transmembrane *albumin concentrations, acid -base balance, hydrostatic and oncotic pressure gradients, oxygen-carbon dioxide concentration gradients*, as well as *ATP and calcium ion concentrations* along membrane surfaces. When the sum aggregate of all these influences cause the glycocalyx to feedback loop back to mitochondria to increase energy combustion, they are separately sending messages back to the continuous outer membrane to increase exposure to certain adhesion and rolling receptors. Al of this choreography enables a sequenced immune arsenal trafficking into the interstitial space through capillary cell transmembrane channels and its gap junctions.

When feedback loop messages go in reverse to decrease immune arsenal trafficking into the interstitial space, the glycocalyx will be messaged to reconfigures its mesh infrastructure and reduce receptor attachment exposures. When this occurs, momentum builds for feedback loop messaging to reduce outer membrane permeability to trafficking while swinging mitochondria combustion to nitric oxide. Immune arsenal trafficking through capillary cell outer membranes decreases as gap junctions close, outer membrane voltage gradients increase, and adhesion receptors recede back into membrane infrastructure. In this manner the glycocalyx holds considerable sway over the capillary cell outer membrane CAM (adhesion molecule) system in affecting inflammatory momentum into or out of the interstitial space.

Glycocalyx sway falls apart when chronic interstitial space momentum blocks the capillary cell dance. In this setting, the glycocalyx mesh thins, the receptor network is silenced and voltage gradients decrease. The glycocalyx becomes much less responsive to interstitial space or end organ signaling. These changes portend a dark interstitial space and poor capillary cell health. The finger ultimately gets pointed back to capillary cell mitochondria and their failure to swing combustion back to nitric oxide. In reality the real problem is an overloaded interstitial space with vascular inflammatory free radicals.

A healthy glycocalyx has a net *negative charge,* which has implications that involve its electromechanical (EM) gradient. Varying the glycocalyx EM gradient nuances further gating of immune arsenal trafficking. When certain proinflammatory mediators, such as *VEGF* (vascular endothelial growth factor) and *TNF (tumor necrosis factor)* interact with the glycocalyx, the EM gradient gets reduced meaning there is less of a negative charge. This increases glycocalyx permeability to a potentially broader spectrum of inflammatory mediators, thereby expanding inflammatory intent entering the interstitial space. If VEGF or TNF exposures decrease the EM gradient, inflammatory dispersal increases exponentially to potentially become more random. This becomes a seed to the induction of rebel immune arsenal eventually bypassing the capillary cell feedback loop communication system.

Capillary and Endothelial Cell Basement Membrane

In contrast to the luminal glycocalyx, on the opposite (abluminal) side of the capillary and abutted up against the interstitial space and end organ cell outer membranes lies the *basement membrane.* The basement membrane can be radically different from one end organ to the next depending on how the end organ functions. In this regard it can be r more of a full blown barrier support (brain), a filtering membrane (kidney) or more like a sieve (liver sinusoid).

The basement membrane is also vulnerable to vascular inflammatory free radical attachment, which over time becomes the linchpin to chronic inflammation. As the basement membrane thickens from proinflammatory debris, the mechanics of interstitial space sanitation and end organ intimacy decrease. Basement membrane thickening can occur anywhere from the largest artery to the smallest capillary but its proinflammatory effects on the interstitial space and end organ they serve are universal

The corresponding figure below demonstrates a generic looking basement membrane of a capillary cell. Like the glycocalyx it is a separate functioning endothelial cell outer membrane distinct from the continuous outer membrane. The basement membrane has specialized infrastructure to nuance specific end organ requirements. It becomes the primary communicating membrane of the endothelia with the interstitial space and end organ.

Since different end organs have vastly different functions, the capillary cell basement membrane has adjusted to accommodate these differences. Basement membranes can have varying levels of *thickness, gaps, pores, receptors* and *voltage gradients.* Generally, a thinner basement membrane with more gaps and a reduced voltage gradient will increase risk to the interstitial space for more adverse exposures from blood plasma. This is seen in spades with the capillary cell in the liver sinusoid. To counterbalance this risk, the capillary cell employs an array of interstitial space helper or mesenchymal cells. Together these cells patrol the interstitial space of Disse within the liver sinusoid and provide an extra arm of protection from potential exposures to infectious agents, cancer cells or other toxins.

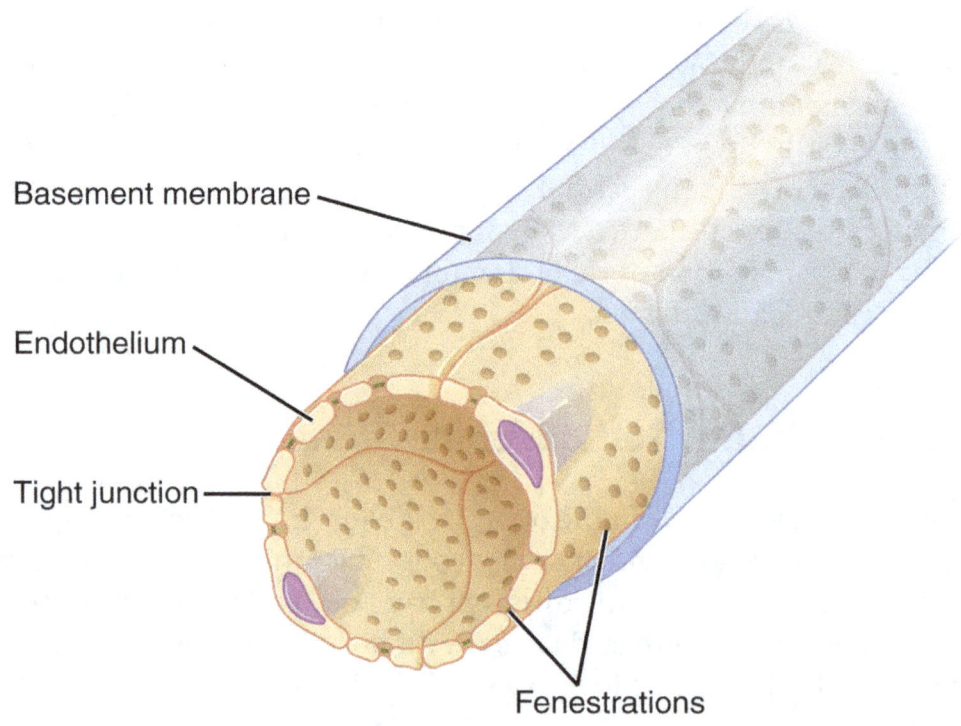

Basement membrane

Endothelium

Tight junction

Fenestrations

Infrastructure of Capillary-Cell Outer Membranes

The infrastructure of the basement membrane is usually composed of interlocking glyco and lipoproteins that include *collagen IV, fibronectin, laminin, chondroitin sulfate and heparan sulfate proteoglycan, perlecan, and entacti*. Within the capillary cell continuous outer membrane scaffolding are *laminin* and *collagen IV polymers* which assist in the stereotaxic display *integrin* and selectin (CAM) adhesion receptors. When activated by protein kinase switches, these infrastructure proteins will twist and bend to expose different adhesion receptors which then can attach a specific cytokine or white blood cell from the blood plasma. In conjunction with other membrane proteins, such as *thrombospondin,* they cascade an immune arsenal choreography which is further nuanced by adjustments to voltage gradients, pores, vesicles, transport channels and gap junction width.

The twisting and bending mechanics of capillary cell outer membrane infrastructure is in a constant state of flux. Depending on interstitial space inflammatory momentum or calls from the end organ for more oxygen and nutrient, outer membrane infrastructure responds in kind to increase or decrease receptor exposures, voltage gradients or even the basement membrane surface area to juxtapose to those of the end organ. The infrastructure coordination places all three endothelial surface membranes on the same page, which is to either expand or contract immune arsenal into the interstitial space or expand or contract oxygen and nutrient delivery to the end organ.

When chronic inflammation masterminds feedback loop control away from the capillary cell, the glycocalyx thins and the basement membrane thickens. This coincides with a loss of receptor volume, voltage gradient responsiveness and capacity of infrastructure to bend, twist and expose receptors. As capillary cell outer membranes lose capacity to function, mitochondrial volumes decrease and feedback loop channels become pirated by chronic inflammation. Choreography is now blown and replaced by random immune arsenal entry, which becomes a perfect gateway to an alternative feedback loop communication system.

Can basement membranes thin and glycocalyx thicken to their more youthful appearance? This will depend on the how well capillary cells can resume dancing after free radical have been reduced within interstitial spaces.

Capillary Cell Continuous Outer Membrane

Enclosing the endothelial and capillary cell cytoplasm is the *continuous outer membrane.* This mother of all membranes serves as a go- between as it mediates signaling between the interstitial space, basement membrane, glycocalyx and blood plasma. It is replete with a host of different receptors, on-off switches and pores that in aggregate execute permeability adjustments while also pacing feedback loop signaling momentum throughout the interstitial space and back towards their mitochondria. Part of it feedback loop power it the capacity to adjust the shape of the capillary cell from flat to oval to hasten or slow the pace of trafficking adjustments. Going form flat to oval opens the gap junction orifice and widens the channel enabling an increased pace of immune arsenal entry. The continuous outer membrane also has its own sets of pores, which vary by size, inherent voltage gradients and diaphragm thickness. The continuous outer membrane (COM) can further affect permeability by adjusting their voltage gradients and activating vesicle and transcellular transport through the capillary cell by endocytosis (moving molecules into the interstitial space or exocytosis (moving them into blood plasma). In this manner, the capillary cell continuous outer membrane becomes the trafficking guru and expert choreographer.

The continuous outer membrane is also responsible for maintaining the optimal homeostasis within the capillary cell that includes the regulation of fluids, electrolytes, proteins, and the various pressure gradients that occur between their cytoplasm, organelles and outside of the cell. This requires constant attention to albumin concentrations on both sides of the membrane as well as how albumin is pulled into the interstitial space with inflammatory breach. Finally, much of this outer membrane push and pull is orchestrated by additional mechanics that involve *diffusion, facilitated diffusion or active transport.*

The continuous outer membrane is strategically bolted to *actin-myosin fibrils,* which in the presence of mitochondrial release of calcium ions and ATP-energy, slide (contract) to dramatically reconfigure the capillary cell morphology. Actin-myosin contraction provides the capillary cell with the capacity to become oval which paces immune arsenal entry into the interstitial space. This has substantial bearing to the success or failure of inflammatory breach elimination.

When capillary cells go oval, it strongly incentivizes feedback loops that signal mitochondria to combust more energy and release calcium ions. The feedback loops are initiated through continuous outer membrane *c AMP* and *kinase on-off switches,* which chain react cascades of outer membrane adjustments leading to increases in permeability and trafficking of immune arsenal. Thus the flux of the COM becomes dependent on interstitial space signaling, energy, calcium ions, cAMP and the families of kinase switches. The execution then depends on the health of outer membrane receptors, membrane infrastructure and mitochondrial volumes. When vascular inflammatory free radicals and other perpetrators of inflammatory breach are contained, membrane cAMP increases, protein kinases are switched off, calcium and ATP accumulate in the cytoplasm and subsequently feedback to mitochondria to swing combustion to nitric oxide. With excessive free radical or foreign perpetrators impinging the interstitial space and basement membranes, the opposite occurs.

If interstitial space sanitation is optimal, all continuous outer membrane switches, receptors and infrastructure operate as a seamless unit as they solidify feedback loop control of the interstitial space and secure effective refurbishment of capillary cell outer membranes and infrastructure. This powerful and dynamic feedback loop system, generated by capillaries and endothelial cells, also paces and stems refurbishment of interstitial space allies, the mesenchymal and end organ cells. Doing so optimizes future choreography in response to interstitial space breach. The combinations of all these COM check and balance trafficking techniques coordinate choreography which increases precision of the immune arsenal response.

Let's summarize in part the COM mechanics for pacing molecules into and out of the interstitial space;

- *Kinase on-off* switches, linked to cAMP, calcium and energy, initiate trafficking momentum.
- A flexing of infrastructure proteins to expose different adhesion receptors for attachment.
- *Pores* of varying sizes, voltage gradients, and diaphragms, can further nuance the type and pace of immune arsenal delivery into the interstitial space.
- *Pits,* found within capillary cell outer membranes of certain capillary cells can extract bulky nutrient from blood plasma.
- Fluxing *electromechanical (EM) voltage gradients,* which provide additional momentum to permeability mechanics to support either a relaxing or restrictive fence to the movement of blood plasma constituents.
- Energy driven *transport vesicles and trans cellular channels,* which help traffic and pace immune arsenal, albumen, or other bulky molecules into or out of blood plasma and the interstitial space.
- Elaborate displays of different *adhesion and rolling protein receptors (CAMs)* that attach specific inflammatory mediators (white blood cells, cytokines) of the immune arsenal. They in turn can be rolled to gap junction orifices or mobilized to enter vesicles or transport channels.
- Through *actin and myosin fibril* contraction and relaxation, the capillary cell outer membrane can reconfigures from flat, which services the end organ, to oval, which expands immune arsenal for the management of interstitial space breach.
- Utilizing *diffusion, passive diffusion and active transport* to optimize fluid, electrolyte, protein and gas movement across COM surfaces

The sophisticated mechanics of capillary cell outer membrane flux of permeability make them the controlling "portal of exit and entry" of blood plasma constituents into and out of the interstitial space. As the capillary continuous outer membrane fluxes permeability it consolidates messaging with the basement membrane and glycocalyx to provide further trafficking momentum. All this goes for naught when COMs get sick from too much interstitial space inflammation. As COMs pseudocapillarize, mitochondrial volumes evaporate, as the glycocalyx thins and basemen membranes thicken. All of this blocks the capillary cell dance, stalls fluxing of outer membrane permeability and encourages random trafficking of immune arsenal into the interstitial space. The space gets darker as it prepares for a rebel immune arsenal coupe of feedback loop signaling control away from the disabled capillary cell.

Let's summarize optimal capillary and endothelial cell COM trafficking:

- In response to an interstitial space inflammatory breach or free radical basement membrane attachment(s), capillary cell outer membranes are signaled to increase permeability to inflammatory mediators entering the interstitial space from blood plasma. This coincides with activation of protein kinase switches, as cAMP levels decrease. Feedback loops chain react to mitochondria calling for calcium ion and ATP release as mitochondria are told to combust more energy.

- In the presence of calcium ions and energy, actin- myosin fibrils contract causing the capillary cell to reconfigure to oval. This widens the gap junction orifice and channel thereby increasing the pace and volume of immune arsenal entry.
- As gap junctions expand, selective CAM receptors are activated to enable attachment and rolling of specific white blood cells and other immune arsenal support as it arrives from blood plasma. Selective receptor exposure seals effective COM choreography.
- Energy driven active transport of additional immune arsenal proceeds through vesicles and transport channels as the capillary cell maintains gas, electrolyte and albumin pressure support on both sides of its outer membranes.
- Activated COM pores catch bulky immune proteins (immunoglobulins) and bud vesicles to accentuate transport process.
- When breach is removed, the process goes in reverse, COM permeability decreases, cAMP levels increase, kinase switches are turned off, calcium and energy accumulate within the cytoplasm and feedback to mitochondria to swing combustion to nitric oxide. Restoration then begins.

In this manner the capillary cell continuous outer membrane uses flux to serve its *two* distinct purposes-interstitial space sanitation while responding to a unique end organ function. Its perfect feedback loop partner in this chain reaction is their mitochondria. The endothelia COM flux becomes the body's fountain of youth.

CAMS

The key piece to the mechanics of capillary COM choreography is the activation and exposure of specific *adhesion receptors* or CAMs. Specific adhesion receptors are exposed on the basis of feedback loop surveillance signaling from the interstitial space. CAMS rotate to become exposed to blood plasma white blood cells or cytokines on the basis of what is called for from interstitial space immune intelligence. When certain kinase switches are activated, COM infrastructure is rotated and certain CAMs exposed.

One set of on-off switches that control CAM activation are the *adhesion kinase family*. One member(s) of this family is *FAK (focal adhesion kinase)*. When focal adhesion kinase is switched on, membrane infrastructure bends to expose a specific CAM. When the desired white blood cell attaches to the CAM, it activates *selectin* receptors, which then roll (guide) the white blood cell to the gap junction orifice. FAK activation requires COM infrastructure response which involves may different moving infrastructure pieces including fragments of *talin, actinin, paxillin, vinculin, tensin, filamin, and zyxin.*

Many different kinds of proinflammatory constituents within or without the interstitial space can activate FAK. Within the capillary cell's cytoplasm one of these constituents is from mitochondrial combustion exhaust (*superoxide, hydroxynitriles*). Outside of the capillary cell cytoplasm other FAK activators include *growth factors (such as VEGF-vasoactive endothelial growth factor), or* other proinflammatory mediators *(histamine, thrombin, and TNF-tumor necrosis factor).*

Depending on what controls interstitial space feedback loops (chronic inflammation or the capillary cell), will determine whether FAK activation works for or against interstitial space sanitation. When FAK is activated by capillary cells, as part of a sequenced choreography to inflammatory breach, FAK activation occurs for the right reason. When FAK activation is hijacked by rebel immune arsenal through the induction of inappropriate levels of histamine, thrombin or VEGF among others, the response it generates supports chronic interstitial space inflammation and will be used for darker purposes.

Two other important COM kinase switch families are the *SRC (non-receptor protein kinases)* and *Rho (RhoA, RAC, Cdc-42)* families. These membrane proteins help to facilitate energy transfer to capillary outer membranes and become critical to the active transport of immune arsenal via vesicles or transcellular channels. These kinases facilitate uncoupling of phosphorus from either ATP or GTP to thereby release energy. This allows COM to option energy where it is needed, whether to mobilize immune arsenal or to further support different membrane pumps and voltage gradients.

It takes a village of different protein kinase on-off switches on capillary cell outer membrane surfaces to execute immune arsenal trafficking while chain reacting feedback loops to mitochondrial combustion. All of these feedback loops get scrambled when these switches are influenced by deceptive cytokine messages received rebel immune arsenal. In other words, the capacity to choreograph is only as good the intelligence the capillary cell COM receives.

The Liver-Endothelial-Capillary Cell Partnership: The Albumin Effect

Albumen in the most abundant blood plasma protein in humans as 15 grams per day is produced daily by normal functioning adult livers. Albumen nuances endothelial and capillary cell membrane permeability in many different ways. Chief among them is how it affects pressures on membrane surfaces, specifically *oncotic* and *hydrostatic* pressures. The oncotic pressure effect on a membrane surface occurs when there is a greater concentration of albumin on one side of the membrane compared to the other. The side with the higher concentration of albumin will passively (without the use of energy) *pull* liquid and electrolytes (sodium, potassium, chloride, phosphate) across membrane surfaces thereby *dehydrating* the space on the opposite side of the membrane. The dehydrating effect of albumin can be critical to expanding and contracting interstitial space edema fluid. With a serious interstitial space inflammatory breach albumin is pulled into the interstitial space, bringing water and electrolytes with it to cause a relative dehydration of the capillary cell.

While some level of edema may be necessary to optimally combat inflammatory breach, it can become excessive. Increased edema fluid impairs capillary end organ gas exchange which could severely compromise end organ function as it becomes prone to hypoxia. A well -known example is the edema fluid that accumulates within the interstitial spaces of lung alveoli linked to pneumonia. The fluid impairs the capacity to exchange oxygen and carbon dioxide to such as degree that worsening hypoxia, electrolyte disturbances and pneumonia often result.

The opposite occurs when the interstitial space is allowed to "dry out". Drying out occurs when albumin concentrations increase within the capillary cell. This can ripple anti-inflammatory cascades that include the pulling of immune arsenal and other inflammatory debris out of the interstitial space. This albumin pulling effect helps cement interstitial space cleanup and contributes to the recycling of inflammatory residues, as albumin often piggybacks cytokines and other inflammatory residues within its bulky infrastructure. Once these residues are pulled into the bloodstream they can be retrieved, permanently removed or recycled in the liver, lymph, bone marrow, spleen and kidney.

Thus endothelial and capillary cells *regulate fluid shifts* into and out of the interstitial spaces of end organs through albumen shifts from one side of the COM to the other. The ramification of albumin homeostasis by capillary cells, not only involves the expansion and contraction interstitial space edema in response to inflammatory breach, but also impacts COM voltage gradients. When albumin homeostasis between the liver and capillary cells is optimal, capillary cell outer membranes are more likely to flux their permeability robustly enabling a better likelihood of successful response to inflammatory breach.

In addition to co- participating in oncotic and hydrostatic homeostasis within the interstitial space, albumin can *chaperone* delivery of fatty acids and other molecules from blood plasma while also assisting in the opposite direction through the removal of cytokines and inflammatory debris. In this manner, albumin functions like a truck, delivering supplies in one direction and removing inflammatory debris in the other.

This occurs when albumin exposes negative or positive charges in its molecule. As it does, it will *vagabond* different fatty acids to catch a ride into the capillary cell or interstitial space space where they can be released. Once released the re exposed charges can be utilized to pick up inflammatory debris in the opposite direction. The vagabond effect does not require energy to facilitate. These albumin "special deliveries" into the capillary cell can include essential fatty acids (fatty acids that cannot be manufactured in cells) or even antioxidants. Many of these transported fatty acids are utilized by the capillary cell when rejuvenation occurs during nitric oxide combustion.

Gap Junctions

Fundamental to choreographed immune arsenal trafficking into interstitial spaces is the gap junction *collection, categorization and dispersal* of white blood cells in a process known as *diapedesis*. Gap junctions are found between all cells, but in endothelial and capillary cells that have specialized to manage immune arsenal dispersal into interstitial spaces. They expand or contract their width, depending on capillary cell change in configuration from flat to oval, thereby providing rate control of white blood cell and cytokine entry into the interstitial space.

Within gap junctions is an intricate array of different check points composed of canals and bridges that help further navigate the pace of specific white blood cell movement. In this manner some cells are held up while others are allowed to flow through the gap junction channel. Decisions to stop or go white blood cell movement receive input from several sources along the route including signals from capillary cell cytoplasm provided by interspersed *connexin* bridges. Gap junctions also have specialized adhesion receptors at their orifice known as *cadherin receptors.* These different receptors, when exposed through stereotaxic shifts, facilitate the entry of a specific blend of white blood cells into the gap junction. As such cadherin receptors play an important role in further nuancing white blood cell choreography into the interstitial space. Capillary cell gap junctions can vary from one end organ to the next, as they can be tightly compacted (blood brain barrier) to be more restrictive in immune arsenal dispersal, or they can be loosely arranged (liver sinusoid) for more liberal movement.

Regardless of whether gap junctions are loose or tightly compacted, they respond similarly to an interstitial space inflammatory breach. For a given type and quantity of inflammation, capillaries are signaled to convert their outer membrane configuration from flat to oval, reconfigure exposures of specific adhesion receptors and adjust the width of the gap junction channel to accommodate nuanced white blood cell entry into the interstitial space.

Capillary and endothelial cell gap junctions consist of four distinct compartments that function as a collection of interlocking canals. In aggregate they systematically control the type and pace of different white blood cell trafficking. These compartments include an *adherens junction* (AJ), *tight junction* (TJ), the *gap junction channel*, and *inter endothelial junctional proteins* (IEJ proteins). Included in the mix are *connexins, which* as discussed previously are interlocking bridges between endothelial cells that signal gap junction white blood cell mobilization from the capillary cytoplasm.

Adherens junction, or *AJs,* are part of the *cadherin receptor complex* that compose the gap junction orifice. When different AJ receptors are exposed and activated through combinations of membrane stereotaxic shifting and protein kinase switches (including FAK) they attach incoming rolled white blood cells for entrance into the gap junction. Hence, AJ receptors become part of the capillary cell choreography download that enables specific white blood cells entrance into the interstitial space. As such AJs are one crosscheck, in a series of crosschecks that become a gate keeper to white blood cell entrance in the interstitial space staging area. When AJ receptors are activated, they affect applicable membrane voltage gradients, as they signal feedback loops back to actin-myosin fibrils to slide thereby widening the gap junction orifice and channel.

A misstep in AJ handling of white blood cell entry into the gap junction, such as accepting the wrong white blood cell for a given inflammatory breach, can chain react a series of trafficking mistakes that can become difficult to compensate for. Besides enabling passage to the wrong white blood cell, it can trigger white blood cell pacing mistakes or enable other immune arsenal, such as platelets of clotting factors, inappropriate entrance. This is more likely to occur when the interstitial space is embroiled in chronic inflammatory preoccupation. In these situations, the gap junction orifice and channel eventually break down form pseudocapillarization (lost cadherin receptors, ineffective connexin exchanges, reduced electromechanical gradients, and lost gap junction infrastructure. When gap junctions fail, random white blood cell entrance into the interstitial space becomes flagrant and their rebellion spurs the alternative signaling feedback loop system employed by the chronic inflammatory matrix to seize control of the interstitial space. Of course all this proinflammatory momentum is fueled by vascular inflammatory free radical preponderance within the interstitial space.

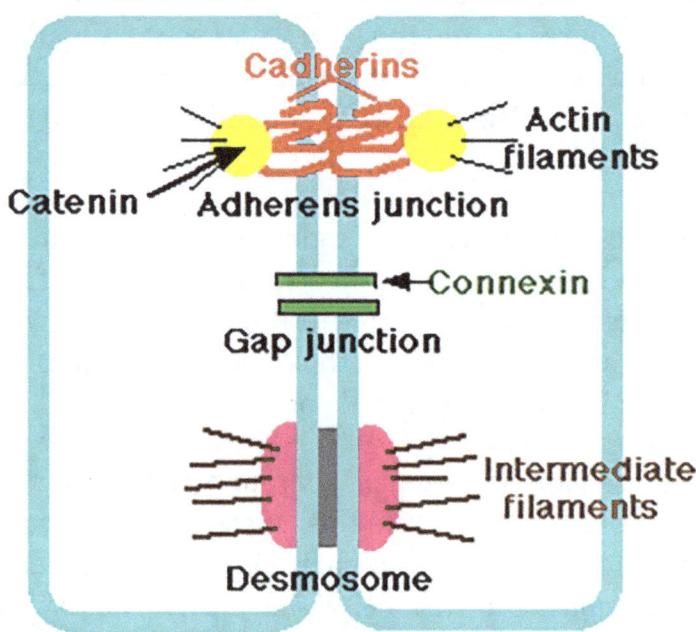

The figure below depicts a gap junction between capillary cells. Displayed are the cadherins receptors at the gap junction orifice which is adjoined to the adherens junction. After choreographed white blood cells pass through the adherens junction, they encounter a bottleneck, known as the tight junction (TJ) (not depicted in the figure). TJs form a tight ring to slow the pace of entry into the gap junction channel. The TJ bottleneck is nuanced through the effects of *claudins, occludins and JAMS (junctional adhesion molecules)*. These different receptors further assist in the selection and pacing of specific white blood cell movement through the gap junction channel. JAMS act as a homing device, as it signals back to the luminal capillary cell continuous outer membrane to enable exposure of specific sets of CAMs for specific white blood cell attachments. Blocking the capability for TJ-JAMS signaling of the luminal COM CAMs becomes a primary target for a more random display of white blood cell entrance into the interstitial space.

In the figure below, the *gap junction channel* (GJ) is the main thoroughfare for white blood cell entrance into the interstitial space. White blood cell movement is paced primarily by expanding or contracting the gap junction orifice and channel width while secondarily affecting movement from effects of the TFJ bottleneck and junctional adhesion proteins. Unlike TJ or JAMS, the gap junction channel membrane surfaces are electric neutral, meaning they don't effect trafficking from changes in voltage gradients.

IEJ proteins (inter-endothelial junctional proteins) are found in both tight and adherins junctions and further nuance trafficking through *PECAM-1 (platelet endothelial cell adhesion molecule. When PECAM-1 is activated, it* blocks certain white blood cell access (neutrophil) to the gap junction channel. Tight junction PECAM-1, claudin, occludin and JAM receptors help to refine the pace and specificity of white blood cell and cytokine choreography as they travel through the gap junction channel.

When chronic inflammation is bearing down on the interstitial space, all of the nuanced choreography mechanics within the gap junction break down, enabling the infusion of more random displays of white blood cells entering the interstitial space staging area. As their concentrations increase they can't help but provide signaling momentum that nurtures an alternative feedback loop communication system that gets superimposed over that of the disabled capillary cell. This darker communication system cascades further proinflammatory momentum which includes a random trafficking of white blood cells and cytokines through the gap junction. The biases extend to enabling the entrance of the wrong white blood cells, as well as the delivery of excessive clotting factors and activated platelets. Coupled with misguided immunoglobulins and the stage is set for a chronic inflammatory coupe that eventually hatches plans for scarring, cancer, thrombosis, autoimmune disease and infections.

Interleukins are inflammatory cytokines that are released from white blood cells. As more random displays of white blood cells enter the gap junction and are dispersed into the interstitial space, their awkward and inappropriate interleukin release becomes the calling card for unintended purposes. As these misguided interleukins disseminate increasingly ineffective messages about inflammatory intent, chain reactions of proinflammatory interstitial space momentum will result. As this is occurring, with capillary cell outer membranes effectively hijacked by the momentum of false messages, it remains hopelessly stuck in increased trafficking mode as their mitochondria combust more energy, without much nitric oxide counterbalance. As superoxide exhaust increases, the trap is set for the capillary cell to succumb from its own combustion toxicity, as superoxide crosslinks and renders DNA increasingly ineffective. Disease venues, fatigue, pain and an aging catharsis will appear almost as if overnight.

Protein Kinase On-Off Switches and the cAMP Feedback Loop

The bending and twisting of capillary cell outer membrane infrastructure to expose different cadres of CAM receptors, initially involves feedback loops signals calling for protein kinase switches to be activated. These different kinase switches are families of different protein and tyrosine kinases that initiate chain reactions which facilitate increases in outer membrane trafficking of immune arsenal. These switches respond to increasing levels of calcium ions at the membrane surface and decreasing concentrations of cAMP (cyclic adenosine monophosphate).

Calcium ions affect capillary cell outer membranes in several ways. First, they decrease sodium and potassium membrane pumps which bias reductions in membrane voltage gradients. Second, they increase actin-myosin sliding(contraction) which reconfigures the capillary cell morphology. Third, along with ATP, facilitate active transport processes across capillary outer membranes. The surge in outer membrane calcium ions comes primarily from their release from the mitochondrial matrix and adjacent smooth endoplasmic reticulum. It coincides with activation of mitochondrial energy combustion and ATP synthase at cytochrome V.

CAMP levels at the outer membrane increase when interstitial space inflammatory breach has been contained and is approaching elimination. Now feedback loops signal from the interstitial space staging area call for a sharp reduction in immune arsenal. As capillary cell outer membrane cAMP re-accumulates, protein kinase switches are turned off and calcium ions and ATP levels increase within the cytoplasm to where they feedback to mitochondria to swing combustion to nitric oxide. This becomes the *rejuvenating swing,* as capillaries restore their infrastructure while stemming similar restoration projects to mesenchymal and end organ cells. As nitric oxide is produced by capillaries, the gas relaxes downstream arteriole smooth muscle thereby enabling increases in blood flow and oxygen delivery to the capillary bed and corresponding end organ. This invariably increases end organ capacity to function as more oxygen delivery means more energy production. Capillary cell outer membrane cAMP and protein kinase switches are powerful tools that can chain react momentum of immune arsenal entry into the interstitial space staging area. When they are hi-jinxed by chronic inflammation, the wrong immune arsenal enters the interstitial space dooming successful breach removal.

CHAPTER 11

WHAT CAPILLARY CELLS ARE TRAFFICKING

Neutrophils

Circulating white blood cells (leukocytes), interleukin - 6 and platelets, are often first line responders to an inflammatory breach within interstitial spaces of end organs. Except for cases of trauma, the initial response should be to signal efforts to *contain* the breach and *expand* inflammation in preparation to eliminate it. The first type of white blood cell to poke its way into the interstitial space is usually the *neutrophil*.

When signaled, circulating neutrophils attach to specific capillary cell outer membrane CAM (adhesion) receptors, and then are rolled by selectin receptors to the gap junction orifice. Once there, they are inherited by cadherin receptors which enable entrance into the gap junction. Once there they make their way through numerous check points within the gap junction channel. In the channel they are selected and paced by different receptor proteins to increase or decrease mobilization into the interstitial space staging area. The pace of delivery to the staging area is influenced by the number of COM-CAM receptors, the width of the gap junction orifice, and the cross talk that occurs within the gap junction enabling choreographed transport.

Upon their arrival in the interstitial space staging area, choreographed neutrophils are programmed to hone in on the offending free radical, particle, cell or infectious agent. Their job is to sacrifice themselves to contain and disable the inflammatory breach, while at the same time, releasing cytokine granules which preempt further instructions for breach containment or immune arsenal expansion. These granules signal intelligence back to capillary cell outer membranes as well as other interstitial space white blood cells and mesenchymal cells to help choreograph the next steps in breach removal.

When neutrophils release their granules they usually expand the inflammatory response. This means that as the die they transition deployment of the next several waves of immune arsenal response, whose singular purpose is to eliminate the breach. In this manner the release of granules by neutrophils parlays effective intelligence improving the precision in capillary cell choreography for the next steps in breach removal. When the immune arsenal response is clicking the initial steps improves the performance of the next steps, thereby providing increased momentum to breach removal.

Lymphocytes

As the interstitial space inflammatory response matures other white blood cells (B and T cell lymphocytes) are often required to complete the mission. These different and highly specialized cells come from a variety of different location including lymph glands, spleen, and bone marrow. These cells also attach and roll on capillary cell outer membranes to eventually enter the gap junction channel, where they are further nuanced before entering the interstitial space staging area. Unlike neutrophils which contain and disable breach, lymphocytes affect breach *elimination*. As they sacrifice themselves to affect breach elimination, they too release additional lymphokines which provide invaluable intelligence back to capillary cell outer membranes and mesenchymal cells as to the next step(s).

The release of lymphokines (lymphocyte cytokines) does two things. First, they can directly *assault* the inflammatory breach and second they can signal for additional support. In this manner, released lymphokines effectively transition the next stage of choreography. As they feedback to capillary cell outer membranes, they will invoke adjustments in permeability that enable greater precision in eliminating inflammatory breach. The mechanics involve the usual capillary cell outer membrane mechanics; exposures of different CAMs for specific immune arsenal attachments, mobilization to the gap junction, and adjustments in outer membrane voltage gradients, pore exposures, and transport channels.

If capillaries stay the course and maintain control of immune arsenal choreography, the inflammatory breach becomes more likely to be eliminated. If chronic inflammation is in control of the inflammatory response, there is likely a preponderance of vascular inflammatory free radical fuel within the interstitial space and breach outcomes are often adverse to the interstitial space and end organ.

The Different Families of Immune Arsenal

The movement of inflammatory mediators into interstitial spaces to nurture sanitation and optimize homeostasis involves an elaborate choreography of sequenced *white blood cells, platelets, complement, clotting factors, immunoglobulins, various cytokines and growth factors*. For best results, the inflammatory response is focused on a specific attack from a foreign or toxic molecule with the choreography managed by capillary cells. When purposed correctly, inflammatory breach is exposed and eliminated completely, the interstitial space sanitation restored, and the capillary cell pivot and swing dance maintained. Any bungling of these steps that result in surpluses or deficiencies of any of the above immune constituents, and rogue momentum builds towards chronic interstitial space inflammation.

The key to effective immune arsenal expansion and contraction into interstitial spaces is the capillary cell outer membrane permeability pivot and mitochondrial combustion swing dance. When the dance is robust the execution of effective immune arsenal expansion and collapse from the interstitial space after breach is exposed and eliminated becomes more likely. It turns out that effective capillary outer membrane function is wholly dependent on its mitochondrial combustion partner and visa-versa.

It takes the right amount of feedback loop signaling from capillary outer membranes to adjust their permeability and the correct amount of energy combustion from mitochondria to execute effective immune arsenal expansion and contraction from the interstitial space. The swing form energy to nitric oxide combustion is just as important as nitric oxide to energy. To little or too much of each and there is accumulation of toxic exhaust and the risk of ineffective energy production or replacement of worn out parts. As such, the robust capillary cell pivot and swing dance sanitizes the interstitial space, rejuvenates the capillary cell infrastructure all while protecting the best interests of its mesenchymal and end organ cell partners. A few misplaced lymphocytes, cytokines, immunoglobulins, complement or platelets, coupled with abundant vascular inflammatory free radical fuel, and chronic inflammation will inevitably grip the interstitial space.

Inflammatory Mediators: Pro or Anti-Inflammatory or Both

Inflammatory mediators, depending on what control s the dynamic of the interstitial space can be pro or anti –inflammatory. Said differently, they can work for or against the best interests of the end organ. Inflammatory expansion of immune arsenal into the interstitial space can be viewed as anti-inflammatory if properly choreographed by capillary cells for a specific purpose. In contrast, if immune arsenal trafficking has become more random and fueled by abundant vascular inflammatory free radicals, immune mistakes compound and signaling feedback loops within the interstitial space are replaced by rogue interests.

In other words, an immune arsenal response to inflammatory breach could begin as *anti-inflammatory,* but with the budding of cascading immune errors, becomes muddled, mistake prone and *proinflammatory.* Regardless of what immune arsenal is designed to do, it can become proinflammatory based on prevailing feedback loops cascades within the interstitial space and how they impact the capillary cell outer membranes. When the prevailing feedback loops block purposed intent to remove inflammatory breach, the interstitial space goes into proinflammatory free fall as the capillary cell dance goes into hibernation. Disease venues populate and pain, fatigue and aging accelerate.

Based primarily on lifestyle choices and to some extent on the genetics we inherit, we foster *our inflammatory fate and the disease venues that result. Depending on the poison we choose, sugar, trans fats, drugs, alcohol, tobacco, polluted air, or couch potato we enable enough proinflammatory fuel within our interstitial spaces throughout our bodies to propagate chronic inflammatory outcomes.*

The corresponding table below highlights potential proinflammatory tailspins that can occur within interstitial spaces when capillary cell lose control of choreography. On the left side are potential inflammatory messages from white blood cells to capillary and mesenchymal cell outer membranes. In the right column, are proinflammatory signals that originate from activated platelets. When white blood cells or platelets within interstitial spaces come "under the influence" of rebel feedback loop signals generated by rogue influences of chronic inflammation, their released messages expand inflammation without a focused intent of breach removal. The interstitial space goes into cascading inflammatory disarray, the capillary cell dance is blocked and disease venues will populate. If these cells and their messages are part of a sequenced choreography delivered by capillary cell outer membranes, the opposite will occur. In the table, leukocytes represent neutrophils and other granulated white blood cells (eosinophils, basophils for example) and all classes of lymphocytes.

Different Activation Products Released by White Blood Cells and Platelets that can Expand the Inflammatory Response

Leukocytes	Platelets
Reactive oxygen species Superoxide free radical Hydrogen peroxide free radical	*Reactive oxygen species* Superoxide free radical Hydrogen peroxide free radical
Proteases (reduces proteins) Cathepsin-G Elastase (reduces elastin) Collagenase (reduces collagen)	*Growth factors* Platelet Derived Growth Factor (PDGF) Transforming growth factor (TGF-β) VEGF
Cytokines/chemokines Interleukins(IL-1, IL-2, IL-6, IL-8, IL-12) Interferons Tumor necrosis factor Transforming growth factor-β Monocyte chemotactic factor-1	*Cytokines/chemokines* IL-1, IL-7, IL-8 RANTES (regulated upon activation, normal T cell expressed and secreted) TNF-β
Oxidases-oxidation Myeloperoxidase-(reduces hydrogen peroxide)	*Lipid mediators* Thromboxane A_2 12-hydroxy eicosatetraenoic acid (HETE)
Lipid mediators Leukotrienes specifically B4, C4 Platelet activating factor	*Procoagulants-pro clotting* Thrombin ADT and ATP
Miscellaneous Cationic (positively charged) proteins Histamine VEGF	

This table implies how important it is for all these released inflammatory components to be correctly choreographed. The constituents mosaic an intricate check and cross checking system that cascade chain reactions of additional wavelets of inflammatory response. Each white blood cell and platelet can release multiple signaling messages that nuance net step responses to eventually remove inflammatory breach. When these chain reactions come under darker influences, the opposite will happen.

How Inflammatory Breach Containment Sets up Elimination

In many occurrences, the *initial* signaling from capillary cell outer membranes involves mobilization of circulating *neutrophils* and cytokines, such as *IL-6 (interkeukin-6)*. As neutrophils enter the interstitial space staging area, they hone in on the foreign molecule, sacrifice themselves and release their granules. This not only stuns and disables the invader, but chain reacts signals to the capillary cell outer membranes the formulate intelligence for the next steps in breach removal. These messages call out further reinforcements, which could include additional neutrophils and cytokines for containment or for the addition of *inducer T lymphocytes* into the staging area.

It is primarily within the gap junction that the pace of immune arsenal entry into the interstitial space is aptly controlled. Not only does the gap junction orifice open or close to limit pace of movement, but pace is further nuanced by the checks and balances of AJs, connexin bridges, and other protein receptors within the gap junction that secondarily effect claudin, occludin, PECAM 1 and JAM receptors among others.

As these different white blood cells proceed in sequence into the interstitial space to systematically deconstruct inflammatory breach, they send intelligence that chain reacts what is needed for eventual next step elimination.

How Breach Elimination Sets up Regeneration

It should be recognized that an inflammatory breach could be anything *foreign* that does not belong in the interstitial space or on the basement membrane. This includes all vascular inflammatory free radicals, in some cases end organ waste, as well as bacteria, viruses, parasites, cancer cells, noxious gases and particulates. Each of these entities will require different arrays of immune arsenal for containment and elimination. This makes proper capillary cell choreography even more important.

After interstitial space inflammatory breach has been contained, intelligence from the breach staging area will send signals through different cytokines to sequence entry of *T helper lymphocytes*. These cells focus on *disassembly* of the breach offender. Disassembly breaks up the offender into smaller molecular components. When completed, T helper lymphocytes, will often signal for *monocytes* or interstitial space *macrophages* to enter the staging area. Along with cytokines, immunoglobulins and complement, they facilitate the final phase of breach mop-up. They engulf, digest and catabolize debris (*phagocytosis*) into simple molecular constituents, which can then be recycled (though the liver) or permanently disposed of (through the kidney).

When clean-up nears completion, signals from the last group of mop-up cells tell capillary cell outer membranes to close down further immune arsenal entry. This critical signal decreases capillary cell outer membrane permeability to immune arsenal trafficking which chain reacts feedback loops back to mitochondria to swing combustion to nitric oxide. *Breach elimination* pushes capillary cell rejuvenation through mitochondrial nitric oxide combustion, thereby becoming an important quality assurance parameter for future responses to inflammatory breach.

The all clear signal from monocytes and macrophages at the staging area loops back to capillary cell outer membranes to increase cAMP, turn off protein kinase switches, close the gap junction orifice, and hide CAM adhesion and selectin receptors. These capillary cell outer membrane adjustments are facilitated by how they cause increases in cytoplasmic calcium ions and unused ATP. Calcium ions and ATP feedback to mitochondria for the subsequent combustion swing to nitric oxide. The capillary cell dance goes into full force.

How Capillary Cells Regeneration Proceeds Through the Mitochondrial Combustion Swing

When capillary cell mitochondria shift combustion to nitric oxide, their matrix shifts *acetyl Co A* away from the Krebs cycle, and instead enables mobilization outside of the mitochondria to adjacent *ribosomes and rough endoplasmic reticulum. This shift in acetyl co A from energy combustion to protein synthesis,* becomes the backbone to endothelial-capillary cell regeneration. As damaged or worn out outer membrane protein receptors are replaced, mitochondrial volumes are repleted. Infrastructure including other organelles is also refurbished and nuclear telomeres, which protect chromosomal DNA, are regrown. These processes provide important feedback loops to interstitial space mesenchymal and end organ cells to process similar refurbishment.

As capillary cell nitric oxide driven rejuvenation occurs, the gas relaxes downstream arteriole smooth muscles causing increases in blood flow to upstream capillaries. As blood flow increases to the capillary bed, as part of its permeability adjustment, the capillary cell reconfigures its outer membrane to become flat and expose as much of its basement membrane as possible to the end organ to maximize contact with end organ outer membranes which enhances intimacy, nutrient and oxygen exchanges enabling increased end organ capacity to function.

In addition to enhanced basement membrane exposure to end organ outer membranes, the capillary cell glycocalyx infrastructure and receptors are refurbished which restores its thickness. As the glycocalyx thickens and the capillary cell flattens out, the gap junction orifice narrows to block potential entry of unwanted white blood cell trafficking. When capillary cells rejuvenate, their optimized homeostasis fuels similar paced rejuvenation of the interstitial space, and its allied partners.

A Forgotten White Blood Cell

In addition to neutrophils, inducer and helper T lymphocytes, monocytes and macrophages, a fourth group of white blood cells can also be called to the staging area. *Mast cells* can be considered part of the mesenchymal cell network. When signaled, they migrate to the breach staging area and function similarly to circulating *basophils,* which is another type of granular white blood cell similar to the neutrophil.

With certain types of particulate exposures within interstitial spaces, mast cells release *histamine, a potent inflammatory expander.* Not only does histamine cause rapid expansion of immune arsenal trafficking into the staging area, but it also chain reacts the activation of *bradykinin.* Both histamine and bradykinin working together are dual functioning inflammatory expanders. They cause affected capillary cells to dramatically increase outer membrane permeability to rapidly escalate an interstitial space inflammatory response. The release of mast cell histamine is often seen with sinus and lung particulate exposures, or in some cases, the presence of viruses or bacteria. In some cases, mast cells will partner with another granular white blood cell known as an *eosinophil* to cause an *allergic response* that includes sneezing, nasal congestion, sinus headaches, shortness s of breath and coughing from acute bronchial asthma.

Platelets

The unnecessary introduction of platelets into the interstitial space can have dangerous thrombosis repercussions. When randomly pushed into the interstitial space by rebel influences, they can couple with clotting factors to precipitate a *thrombosis.* Thrombosis, regardless of where it occurs, unless being utilized to stop hemorrhage, can be life threatening to the affected end organ. In most cases, thrombosis cuts off blood flow or oxygen delivery to cells and tissues upstream. The larger the blood vessel affected the greater the risk to upstream cell viability. In most cases, thrombosis occurs from the progression of endothelial cell basement membrane thickening and the evolution of obstructive plaque impinging the membrane surface to dangerously narrow the vessel lumen. Platelet activation can also be a part of a lethal muse deployed by the anti-organ as part of a different disease venues that include growing cancers, chronic infections or autoimmune complex diseases.

Abnormal platelet activation is a prime time contributor to the thrombosis double whammy that is caused from progressive downstream large vessel basement membrane thickening, obstructive plaque and progressive lumen narrowing, which compounds capillary cell panic upstream as it scrambles to manage ineffective oxygen delivery and the same proinflammatory influences on its basement membrane. The double whammy puts intense pressure on capillaries that ultimately becomes a no win in solving the end organ oxygen deficit problem.

When large vessel plaque narrows a blood vessel lumen by 90%, blood velocity slows through the narrowing enabling platelets to aggregate, occlude and form the thrombosis. Whether the occlusion affects one large vessel or several smaller ones, the net impact on the end organ is the same, a devastating fracture of functional capacity. In the brain this can be seen when one large stroke paralyzes one side of the body or when several smaller occlusions take out memory and cognitive skills. The double whammy is all about chronic inflammation, and the accumulation of vascular free radicals on basement membrane surfaces up and down the arterial tree, and the abnormal expansion of immune arsenal towards them. As adverse outcomes from thrombosis metastasize the end organ dies a suffocating death as the capillary cell stands by in futility.

Combined with excessive clotting factors and chronic inflammatory disease venues involving cancer or chronic infections, abnormal platelet dispersal can result in a *hypercoagulabilit*y state. In other words, chronic inflammation further impacts end organ function by coupling a disease venue with increased clotting and thrombosis risk. This means the clots can show up in veins in addition to those seen from arterial vessel obstructive plaque. Just like oxygen cutoff, vein clots can also have devastating effects as they migrate and thrombose in veins to cause *emboli*.

In addition, platelets can release their own sets of of platelet derived *VEGF* (vasoactive endothelial growth factor) and *thrombin*. Both expand different mosaics of interstitial space inflammation which further contribute to additional interstitial space clotting biases.

When platelet dispersal and activation within the interstitial space becomes chronic, clotting biases increase and results in a proinflammatory kaleidoscope of thrombosis risk to the end organ. That risk is layered with chain reactions favoring disease venues that include chronic infections, cancers, autoimmune diseases and scarring.

Mesenchymal Cells-Making or Breaking Interstitial Space Sanitation

The loyal right hand to capillary cell choreography in effectively managing interstitial space sanitation is the cadre of different helper cells known as *mesenchymal cells*. This consortium of interstitial space cells forms unique partnerships with both capillary and end organ cells. The different numbers and types of mesenchymal cells will vary from one end organ to the next depending on how the end organ functions and what kinds of at risk exposures are occurring within interstitial spaces. In aggregate mesenchymal cells expand the reach of capillary cell interstitial space surveillance and choreography. They become in effect the capillary cell's "extra set of eyes and ears" as they provide additional intelligence as well as participate in the elimination of inflammatory breach.

Mesenchymal cells can be considered a type of *stem cell,* as their *progenitors* can differentiate into different cell types with different functions. In the liver sinusoid, mesenchymal cells become predominantly *stellate cells and Kupffer cells*. In the skin, they are known as *melanocytes*. In the brain, they compose a *glial* network of cells which include *astrocytes*. In aggregate they link with capillary cells to optimize interstitial space hygiene, which then makes the space favorable to a diverse array of different end organ functions.

Mesenchymal cells communicate with capillary cells by signaling feedback loops. These signals occur as a result of underlying inflammation within the interstitial space and the subsequent demands that arise from fluctuations of end organ function. On the basis of prevailing interstitial space co0ndiitons, signals to the capillary cell outer membranes or the end organ can include the secretion of enzymes, cytokines, growth factors, collagen and amyloid among others, as well as well participating in the actual engulfment (swallowing or phagocytosis) of waste, free radicals, particulates, cancer cells or infectious agents. They also act as reconnaissance experts as they signal back to capillary cell outer membranes to facilitate adjustment of immune arsenal trafficking. When feedback loops between capillary and mesenchymal cells are operational and capillary cell are in control of immune arsenal trafficking choreography, the mesenchymal cell network provides seamless interstitial support for the removal of inflammatory while simultaneously optimizing mechanics of end organ function.

Mesenchymal cells always function best when capillary cells are dancing and vascular inflammatory free radical fuel is minimized within the interstitial space. This serves to minimize the seeding of chronic inflammation which then limits confusion about mesenchymal cell purpose. The more chronically inflamed the interstitial space becomes, the more potential exists for rebel immune e arsenal to feedback loop messages back to mesenchymal cells that scramble purpose. The scrambling eventually works against capillary choreography to increase rather than decrease potential disease venue escalation.

When chronic inflammation hijacks the feedback loop signaling system within the interstitial space, capillary cells don't dance, their outer membranes receptors and mitochondria atrophy, and their feedback loops that control incoming choreography and the affairs of interstitial space immune arsenal and mesenchymal cells lapse. As signaling loops of cytokines are replaced by those of rebel immune arsenal, the mesenchymal cells get caught in the middle and convert allegiance based on prevailing feedback loop control. The weakened capillary cell no longer has the capability to manage signaling operations. The persistent and subversive messages from rogue immune arsenal within the interstitial space, switch inflammatory momentum to increase risk for expansion of disease venues rather fighting them. Mesenchymal cells are brought along for the ride.

The new feedback loop signals run opposite to capillary cell choreography. The switch pushes the mesenchymal cell families within the interstitial space to assist in the building of different disease venues. Combined with a rebel immune arsenal gone bad, the interstitial space pieces have come together to enable expansion of the chronic inflammatory anti-organ outcomes.

Besides the specialized mesenchymal cells found in specific end organ interstitial spaces, what do the other mesenchymal cells look like? Harbored in most end organ interstitial spaces is the *fibroblast*. These cells can be described as large- flat branching cells similar to the stellate cell in the liver sinusoid. When activated, fibroblasts can secrete *collagen, elastin and proteoglycans*. When capillary cell choreography is in control of interstitial space dynamics, these substances are used by assembled immune arsenal to assist in the elimination of inflammatory breach. When fibroblast secretion is under the control of chronic inflammation, these substances can block discovery to promote breach expansion while further undermining communication between disabled capillary and end organ cells. Persistent fibroblast secretion under false pretenses will induce amyloid or fibrous scar tissue. In the liver this chronic inflammatory progression is known as cirrhosis, in the lung, fibrosis, in the kidney, glomerulosclerosis, and in the brain, the various types of dementia, including Alzheimer's disease.

Another type of mesenchymal cell, the *macrophage,* act as recyclers and garbage disposals. They engulf (swallow) and degrade (chemically breakdown) interstitial space inflammatory debris. Unlike monocytes which are circulating lymphocytes that migrate into the interstitial space to perform similar duties, macrophages tend to be more stationary. They function similar to an amoeba as they encircle, engulf and catabolize inflammatory debris. Its capacity to recognize and respond to inflammatory mop-up operations is severely compromised under the auspice of the confusing array of feedback loop signals coming from rogue immune arsenal in the setting of chronic inflammation. This inevitable collapse of the interstitial space will play out in a *pick your poison* of different anti-organ disease venues.

Cytokines-Masters of the Signaling Code

The signaling direction of the complex mosaic of the immune arsenal within the interstitial space is carried out primarily by cytokines. Cytokines represent large families of different proteins that are released from a variety of cells, often as part of a chain reaction, that effect the direction of inflammatory intent within the interstitial space. When properly choreographed, cytokines act to maintain interstitial space homeostasis thereby enabling optimal end organ function. When capillary cell choreography is disabled cytokines become part of the signaling problem, as they show themselves at the wrong time and place. They arise from inappropriate dispersal of rebel immune arsenal into interstitial spaces. Their production and release causes a desynchronizing proinflammatory momentum towards darker interstitial space outcomes.

Most cytokines will induce stimulate or inhibit into the interstitial space the mobilization of white blood cells, platelets, clotting factors and immunoglobulins. In some cases, they become growth factors that increase protein synthesis and cell replication. When properly choreographed by capillaries, cytokines assist in the recruitment of different cells at different times into the interstitial space that eventually push conclusion of an inflammatory breach. They include the trafficking of neutrophils, monocytes, and lymphocytes as well as the activation of macrophages, fibroblasts and platelets. In some cases they facilitate interstitial space entry of clotting factors, complement and immunoglobulins. As such cytokines are central to the feedback loop signaling apparatus used by capillary cells as part of effective choreography or for darker purposes, as chronic inflammation scrambles and confuses their purpose via rogue immune arsenal.

The capillary cell has evolved different receptor packages on their outer membranes to accommodate cytokine responsiveness. At any given moment, cytokines are being released by different cells and engage capillary cell outer membranes to affect permeability trafficking of immune arsenal. For cytokine responsiveness to be effective endothelial and capillary cell outer membranes must demonstrate effective *receptor tone*. This means that their outer membranes must have a full complement of receptors. And they must also have ample support from mitochondria to provide on demand energy and calcium ions or nitric oxide depending on the prevailing conditions within the interstitial space and oxygen- nutrient demands from the end organ.

Cytokine nomenclature can get confusing as there are several different methods of classification. In addition, cytokines can have different names based on different classification systems. A given cytokine can have four different names based on what kind of cell produces them. As an example a given cytokines can be called:

- *Interleukins*-when produced and secreted by T lymphocytes-helper cells
- *Lymphokines*-a more generic term that includes production and secretion from any lymphocyte
- *Monokines*-produced and secreted by monocytes
- *Endokines*-produced by endothelial cells including capillary cells

Cytokines are actually produced by all nucleated cells, which include white blood cells, end organ cells, all endothelia, macrophages, mast cells and other mesenchymal cells. On the basis of the diversity of cytokine origin, it is clear, that capillary cell choreography will enable their effectiveness. Cytokines expression can bias inflammatory expansion or contraction. When in the hands of rebel immune arsenal, cytokine signaling can disrupt competent expansion or contraction of immune arsenal into interstitial spaces.

Another way cytokines are classified is how they function. This can be tricky as cytokines can have different functions based on what cell is producing them and when they arrive at a staging area. For example, tumor necrosis factor (TNF) will have a different effect on an inflammatory breach when produced from an endothelial cell as opposed to a white blood cell. Examples of cytokine classification based on how they function include:

- *Interferons-are* anti-virals, can augment B or T cell lymphocyte responsiveness to the virus.
- *Colony stimulating factors*-affects growth mediators (such as *transforming growth factor-TGF*)
- *Chemokines- (interleulins 1,6,12)* mediate attraction of white blood cells to intended targets

Cytokines can also be classified on the basis of molecular structure:

- *Alpha helix bundle family*-which includes the interleukin-2 (IL-2) families of cytokines-*erythropoietin (EPO)* and *thrombopoietin (TPO)*. Also included in the alpha helix family are IL-10, and interferons
- *IL-1 family*-which includes interleukins(IL) -1 and 18
- *IL-17 family*
- *Cysteine "knot"* cytokine family- which includes *transforming growth factors* 1-3 (TGF 1-3)

The nomenclature for classifying cytokines unfortunately is convoluted, but perhaps is better understood based on what controls the interstitial space and if that controlling influence is working towards inflammatory breach elimination or expansion. In this scenario, it does not matter where the cytokine comes from, or what it does or what its molecular structure is. If the cytokine is part of a sequenced capillary cell choreography, it is likely eliminating inflammatory breach and optimizing interstitial space homeostasis and end organ function. If the controlling influence is chronic inflammation, it will likely expand inflammatory breach, compromise the interstitial space and reduce end organ function.

A common and early responder to an inflammatory breach is interkeukin-6 (IL-6). Depending on the breach, IL-6 concentrations can dramatically increase within interstitial space by several thousand fold in just a few seconds to minutes. In the *initial phase* of an inflammatory response, interleukins 1, 6 and 12 will interact with capillary outer membrane receptors to trigger *uncoupling* or the stereotaxic flipping to expose adhesion receptors. This enables attachment of circulating neutrophil white blood cells and the initial phase of breach containment is well under way.

When IL-6, neutrophils and other early responders are staged into the interstitial space, the acute inflammatory process will expand inflammation. As such, cascades of additional cytokines are produced, interact with capillary cell outer membranes to increase their permeability and in proper sequence, swarm the interstitial space to affect inflammatory breach. Coupled with other arriving immune arsenal, a diverse group of cytokines will interact with capillary cell outer membranes to assist in staging appropriate cascades of next phase immune arsenal arrival into the staging area, similar to how a military force stages an operation to take control of a territory. The mechanics of sequencing immune arsenal will involve the stereotaxic shifting of exposed outer membrane adhesion receptors, the persistent widening of the gap junction orifice, the bottleneck effect of gap junction proteins to pace immune arsenal movement, and the increased presence of outer membrane pores, vesicles and transport channels to assist in immune arsenal mobilization. The fury of increased capillary cell outer membrane permeability will bias reductions in cAMP and membrane voltage gradients, as calcium ions and ATP arrive from mitochondria.

The sum total of the immune arsenal trafficking haul into the interstitial space staging area is finely tuned via the capillary cell controlled feedback loop signaling system. It involves feedback loops from interstitial space immune arsenal, adjacent capillaries, mesenchymal and end organ cells. It will also receive input from downstream endothelia as well as distant end organs. The cytokines represent the signaling apparatus of the feedback loop system. Their release nuances effective capillary cell choreography, thereby creating a greater likelihood of inflammatory breach elimination within the interstitial space. Breach elimination becomes crucial to capillary cell quality assurance as it enables the pivot and swing dance to occur as a result of a downshift in outer membrane permeability. The push to nitric oxide mitochondrial combustion sets up rejuvenation.

As mop-op operations of an inflammatory breach mature, macrophages, T lymphocytes and cytokine (interleukin-10 or IL-10) will provide important feedback loops to capillary outer membranes to decrease permeability and limit trafficking of additional immune arsenal entry into the interstitial spaces. As such the effects of IL-10 on capillary cell outer membranes run contrary to those of IL-6. As outer membrane cAMP levels rise and protein kinases are switched off, adhesion receptors hide within membrane infrastructure, gap unction orifices shrink and voltage gradients increase.

As mitochondrial combustion swings to nitric oxide capillary cell *quality assura*nce to future effectiveness occurs, as protein synthesis is stimulated to repair, replace and replicate anything worn out or dysfunctional. This assures long term viability of the end organ. It also represents the best way to keep chronic interstitial space inflammation, and the disease venues, fatigue, pain and aging it causes, at bay.

The Risk and Benefits of Cytokine Activation

Cytokine release from immune arsenal becomes a liability when interstitial space vascular inflammatory free radicals cannot be contained or eliminated within interstitial spaces. Their dispersal fuels the delivery of rogue immune arsenal into interstitial spaces. When this occurs, the rebel white blood cells release cytokines that have no intention of eliminating inflammatory breach. Their feedback loop momentum instead serves to distract and subvert inflammatory breach removal. As this occurs, a new feedback loop signaling momentum emerges within the interstitial space that hijacks capillary cell outer membranes, subverts mesenchymal cells and renders end organ cells increasingly irrelevant in communicating its interests to their capillary cell partners.

The outcome of this persistent menace to the disabled capillary cell is the blocking of its dance. Outer membranes get stuck in enabling a more random immune arsenal into the interstitial space thereby perpetuating the proinflammatory chain reaction of the darker feedback loop signaling system within the interstitial space. And capillary cell mitochondria are increasingly stuck in energy combustion providing energy for active transport for the trafficking of rebel immune arsenal. The proinfalmmatory momentum makes a mockery of capillary cell function as superoxide generated DNA damage coupled with minimal nitric oxide combustion and cell regeneration block replacement of capillary cell outer membrane receptors (pseudocapillarization) or mitochondrial volumes.

What are considered key pieces to optimal interstitial space homeostasis and end organ function, when released for the wrong reasons and out of sequence, cytokines becomes an interstitial space proinflammatory nightmare.

The sway of proinflammatory momentum is conferred with the inappropriate secretion of interleukins 1,6 and 12, different interferons, TNF and growth factors. Instead of participating in inflammatory breach removal, these different cytokines when released by rebel white blood cells open a flood gate through capillary cells of additional unauthorized and dangerous white blood cells, platelets and immunoglobulins into the interstitial space. This provides a perfect backdrop for proinflammatory chain reactions and chronic inflammatory expansion. In sequence cytokines work in harmony to optimize interstitial space sanitation. Out of sequence, they enable proliferation of disease venues.

The table below is an attempt to arrange cytokines on the basis of where they are produced and their secondary effects on different cellular targets. When part of a principled choreography, they sanitize the interstitial space. The implication is that cytokine effect can be highly *pleomorphic* based on the context of their release. They induce different inflammatory effects based on what controls the interstitial space.

The cytokines of innate immunity

	mass (kDa)	assembly	pdb	source(s)	target(s)
IL1	17	monomer	3O4O	macrophages, endothelia, epithelia	endothelia (↑ coagulation, ↑ inflammation) hepatocytes (↑ acute phase proteins), hypothalamus (↑ fever)
IL18	17	monomer		macrophages	NK lymphocytes (↑ IFN-II γ), T lymphocytes (↑ IFN-II γ)
TNF	17	homotrimer	1TNF, 3ALQ	macrophages, T lymphocytes	endothelia (↑ coagulation, ↑ inflammation) hepatocytes (↑ acute phase proteins), neutrophils (↑ activation), hypothalamus (↑ fever)
IL6	26	homodimer	1P9M (complex)	macrophages, endothelia, T lymphocytes	hepatocytes (↑ acute phase proteins), B lymphocytes (↑ proliferation)
IL15	13	monomer		macrophages	NK lymphocytes (↑ proliferation), T lymphocytes (↑ proliferation
IL12	35/40	heterodimer	1F45 3DUH	macrophages, dendritic cells	Th1 lymphocytes (↑ differentiation), Tc lymphocytes (↑ IFN-II γ), NK lymphocytes (↑ IFN-II γ)
IL23	19/40	heterodimer		macrophages, dendritic cells	T lymphocytes (↑ IL17)
IL27	28/13	heterodimer		macrophages, dendritic cells	Th1 lymphocytes (inhibition and/or differentiation), NK lymphocytes (↑ IFN-II γ),
IL10	18	homodimer	2H24 1Y6K	macrophages, T lymphocytes	macrophages, dendritic cells (↓ IL12)
INF-I (α)	21	homodimer		macrophages	all cells (↑ viral immunity, ↑ MHC class I), NK lymphocytes (↑ activation)
INF-I (β)	25	homodimer	1AU1	fibroblasts	all cells (↑ viral immunity, ↑ MHC class I), NK lymphocytes (↑ activation)
INF-III			3OG4	under study	all cells (↑ viral immunity, ↑ MHC class I), NK lymphocytes (↑ activation)
chemo-kines	8-12	monomer		macrophages, endothelia, fibroblasts, epithelia	phagocyte (↑ migration), B lymphocytes (↑ migration), T lymphocytes (↑ migration), ↑ wound repair

What become clear is how important macrophages are in interstitial space cytokine production. It also makes them an important target for conversion to a darker feedback loop signaling chain. How and when they release cytokines provide critical communication feedback loops to not only endothelial and capillary cells, but also to interstitial space lymphocytes and distant liver cells, where many inflammatory proteins are manufactured. The comingling of cytokine intent makes mesenchymal cells critical to the sequencing path provided by capillary cells which enabling the elimination n of inflammatory breach.

Robert L Buckingham, MD, FACP

Immunoglobulins and Complement: A Trusted Friend or Disruptive Enemy

The immunoglobulin and complement families within the larger family of immune arsenal provide major support to interstitial space inflammatory breach elimination. These circulating proteins are brought into the interstitial space to attach to foreign proteins and inflammatory debris to enable monocytes or macrophages to recognize and phagocytose (engulf or swallow) the newly formed complex. This inflammatory debris could be anything rendered as foreign and include bacteria, virus, particulates, toxins, malignant cells or other large proinflammatory proteins.

When circulating immunoglobulins arrive and are vetted by endothelial or capillary cell outer membranes, some will induce to attach and then be actively transported through the capillary cell and into the interstitial space staging area by vesicles or transport channels. When properly sequenced they attack receptors on foreign proteins deemed hostile to normal interstitial space operations. Once attached, the new entity become like a giant flashing red light known as an *antigen-antibody complex.* Not only does the immunoglobulin disable the foreign protein but it serves as a magnet for *complement proteins* to also attach. Attached complement readies the antigen–antibody complex for monocyte or macrophage engulfment (phagocytosis). Once engulfed, the offender is broken down into basic raw materials and either recycled to the liver or removed as waste in the kidney. Immunoglobulins are an important way of disabling and removing larger foreign proteins, infectious agents or cancer cells. They are keyed into the inflammatory response by immune arsenal and mesenchymal cells feedback loops within the interstitial space to capillary cells, which then vet and sequence them in preparation for transport into the interstitial space.

White blood cells can contain granules and are differentiated into *neutrophils, eosinophils, and basophils based on granule payload.* These cells are part of the early responder network and are responsible for containment of an inflammatory breach. Lymphocytes are also white blood cells and can be further classified into *B or T cells.* As previously discussed T lymphocytes participate as either inducer (early responder to breach) or helper (late responder or elimination of breach) lymphocytes. Circulating immunoglobulins are produced from *plasma cells,* which differentiate from *B lymphocytes or* B cell lymphocytes.

Complement proteins are produced in the liver and circulate in the blood plasma. With an inflammatory breach to an interstitial space, specific immunoglobulins along with complement proteins are signaled to attach and eventually enter the involved interstitial space. In optimal conditions, capillary cells vet, sequence and lockdown a specific set and volume of immunoglobulins and complement thereby bolstering the likely hood of successful breach elimination. Once in the interstitial space, the immunoglobulin should laser like a heat seeking missile to the foreign protein, infectious agent or cancer cell. Once attached, complement proteins follow, which then attracts macrophages or monocytes to engulf the residue. This completes the operation known as *opsonization.* In this sense, *B -plasma cell* lymphocytes, and the immunoglobulins they produce, form a separate immune arsenal operations arm from neutrophil-inducer-helper lymphocytes.

Both arms are critically important to the removal of different types of breach at different times and locations.

Like neutrophils, T inducer and helper lymphocytes, immunoglobulins and complement also team up with cytokines (1,6,12). These cytokines act as early responders to infalmmato0ry breach and are produced and released from mesenchymal and capillary endothelial cells. While these cytokines help to induce an immunoglobulin response, it is how they set up the capillary cell outer membranes to accept a specific immunoglobulin attachment that renders success to interstitial space breach elimination.

The table below summarizes the different immunoglobulins operations. Immunoglobulins *IgG and IgM* circulate within the bloodstream, whereas immunoglobulin *IgA* is found in high concentrations within interstitial spaces of the intestinal tract, lungs and sinuses. Immunoglobulin *IgE* is found primarily in eosinophil granules which are biased to found within interstitial spaces of the skin, sinus and mucous membranes of the nose throat and lungs. Unlike other immunoglobulins, IgE has a strong affinity to bind to mast cells, to release histamine and activate bradykinins, which expands interstitial space inflammation dramatically. This inflammatory response can be life threatening as it increases edema fluid within involved interstitial spaces which can quickly obstruct the airway. IgE release is part of what is known as an *allergic and sometimes anaphylactic response* to an inhaled particulate, drug or bee sting.

The second of two tables below demonstrates how immunoglobulins work. IgG and IgM activate complement to enhance opzonization of a mature *antigen-antibody complex* leading to macrophage and monocyte removal. The other immunoglobulins do *not* attach complement but rather cause the release of other proinflammatory molecules which increase mucous (IgA) production or augment an allergic response (IgE).

Ig class	tissue location/function
IgG	primary immunoglobulin for immunity against invading pathogens in most end organs. Binds to a variety of lymphocytes, monocytes, neutrphils and macrophages.
IgA	mucus – intestinal and respiratory tracts
IgM	early lymphocyte B cell-mediated response to invading pathogens in most end organs
IgD	antigen receptor on B cell lymphocytes
IgE	mast cells – when bound to mast cells, causes release histamines in response to allergens

Immunoglobulin	Relationship to complement	Immune effect
Immunoglobulin G -	complement will attach	Opsonin promotion of phagocytosis. Macrophages, monocytes, neutrophils, and some lymphocytes have receptors for IgG attachment. The attachment of the immune complex (antigen-antibody-IgG complex) facilitates phagocytosis.
Immunoglobulin A -	Secretions - complement will not attach.	IgA antigen-antibody complex can bind to neutrophils and some lymphocytes.
Immunoglobulin M -	complement will attach	IgM binds to some lymphocytes and macrophage receptors. Like IgG, it can form an antigen-antibody complex which can attach to a lymphocyte or macrophages and be engulfed into the cell.
Immunoglobulin D -	No complement fixation	
Immunoglobulin E -	No complement fixation	Binds very tightly to receptors on basophils and mast cells to subsequently cause release of histamine, so involved in allergic reactions

There are at least 30 different complement proteins produced by the liver and circulate within blood plasma. Complement proteins can opsonize a foreign protein with or without immunoglobulin participation. When acting alone, complement produces opsonization through different combinations of *chemotaxis* (attracting lymphocytes, monocytes or macrophages towards the attached foreign protein), *lysis* (rupturing the foreign invader cellular membranes) and *agglutination* (clustering foreign invaders into a group so that they can be more easily recognized and corralled by interstitial space lymphocytes, monocytes and macrophages).

With the emergence of chronic inflammation within interstitial spaces, the effectiveness of immunoglobulins and complement decreases exponentially. This is due primarily to a loss of vetting, sequencing by capillary cell outer membranes, and is further compromised by poor feedback loop signaling from turned mesenchymal cells and rebel white blood cells within the interstitial space. When this happens, immunoglobulins and complement get confused and attach to proteins that are not foreign. In some instances, this involves membrane surfaces of end organs. This critical mistake will chain react cascades of additional immune mistakes as B cell lymphocytes are duped to think the end organ outer membrane protein is actually foreign and should be destroyed. This ends up being a perfect feeder for chronic inflammation to disperse additional disease venues.

The end organ damage from misguide immunoglobulin attachments are known collectively known as collagen vascular diseases. Examples include multiple sclerosis, lupus erythematosus and rheumatoid arthritis but there are many others. As these rogue antigen-antibody complexes gain proinflammatory momentum, the anti-organ will set up the affected interstitial space for cancer, infection scarring or thrombosis.

Thrombin: A Cytokine that can Optimize or Disrupt Anti-Inflammatory Rhythm

Thrombin (known as *factor II*) is a pluripotent circulating molecule, produced in the liver as *prothrombin,* and activated to thrombin by *clotting factors V and X (Stuart Factor).* Thrombin drives the clotting cascade by inducing fibrinogen to become *fibrin.* Fibrin forms a sticky mesh residue which becomes an ideal substrate for platelet adherence. The process forms a clot that is completed by platelets to cause a *thrombosis.* When this process is driven by trauma, cut or open wound, it enables the end organ to potentially stop hemorrhaging and begin to heal. When driven by chronic inflammation in the form of an obstructive plaque, cancer growth or autoimmune complex disease pro clotting biases can work against the end organ to result in reduced oxygen delivery and hypoxic-ischemic events.

Such well known sudden events including heart attacks, strokes, lung (pulmonary emboli) and leg (deep vein thrombosis) clots can be common occurrences in certain disease venues driven by chronic inflammation.

When thrombin attaches to *PAR-1 receptor* (protease activated receptor-1) on the capillary cell outer membrane, a cascading feedback loop signal is generated to mitochondria to release calcium and swing combustion to make energy in preparation for increases in outer membrane trafficking of immune arsenal. Chronic thrombin attachment to the Par-1 receptor becomes a strong blocker of the capillary cell dance as mitochondria get stuck in energy combustion mode. The thrombin –Par-1 attachment is one of many potential mechanisms deployed by chronic inflammation, and fueled by vascular inflammatory free radicals, that prevent the swinging of mitochondrial combustion from energy to nitric oxide and marking the beginning of capillary cell decay from the inside out.

The thrombin-Par-1 activation causes certain outer membrane kinase switches to be switched through the activation of *PKC (protein kinase C)-alpha, Src* (selective tyrosine kinase), and *adenylate cyclase-6.* The ladder enzyme counterbalances the activation of PKC-alpha by causing increases in membrane *cAMP (cyclic adenosine monophosphate).* Adenylate cyclase-6 therefore becomes an important outer membrane counterbalance to biases in outer membrane trafficking of immune arsenal into interstitial spaces. These biases include the migration of pro clotting molecules, all of which becomes part of the chronic interstitial space inflammatory package. Thus thrombin-Par-1 activation, activates certain kinase switches, reduces membrane cAMP levels and biases increases in outer membrane trafficking of immune arsenal into interstitial while simultaneously asking mitochondria to combust more energy to support active transport processes.

With an interstitial space inflammatory breach, signals are sent from lymphocytes and mesenchymal cells to capillary cell outer membranes to increase permeability to immune arsenal, which includes thrombin. As stored calcium ions are released by mitochondria as they combust energy, they like thrombin-Par-1, facilitates activation of protein kinase C alpha (PKC-alpha). In addition to causing reductions in outer membrane cAMP, PKC-alpha cascades activation of *RhoA-GTPase*. RhoA is a small enzyme composed of guanosine triphosphate (GTP), which activates *ROCK (Rho associated protein kinase)*, thereby enabling outer membrane infrastructure to bend and twist to expose specific CAM (adhesion) receptors. ROCK facilitates CAM attachment by the activation of *FAK (focal adhesion kinase)*. Together, these receptors facilitate sequenced immune arsenal entry into the awaiting gap junction, vesicle or transcellular transport channels. Both the thrombin-Par-1 attachment and calcium ions initiate this cascade. Thus the cascade goes something like this: Calcium ions/thrombin-Par-1 receptor activation- activates PKC-alpha and Src while reducing cAMP-activates Rhoa-GTPase-activates ROCK-activates FAK- which then enables endothelial and capillary cell immune arsenal choreography into interstitial spaces.

Activation of the ROCK-FAK switches are key to enhancing outer membrane CAM exposures. Together, they provide a strong feedback loop block to adenylate cyclase-6 induced cAMP production. Therefore, their activation drives persistent increases in permeability of the capillary and endothelial cell outer membrane. In addition the persistent presence of thrombin attachment to Par-1 receptor provides additional impetus to persistently block cAMP production. These blocks to cAMP production blocks the capillary cell dance, increases risks for chronic inflammatory progression within interstitial spaces and becomes the death rattle for capillary cell over combustion of energy, superoxide free radicals and the silencing of membranes and infrastructure.

The FAK switch (focal adhesion kinase) can be a wild card in this proinflammatory cascade, as it can also increase outer membrane c AMP. That is, when inflammatory breach is successfully being eliminated, FAK can be signaled to *inactivate* RhoA-ROCK, and block CAM outer membrane exposures. White blood cell, certain cytokine and other immune arsenal attachments to capillary outer membranes are then blocked, thereby enabling the pivot and swing of the capillary cell dance. With chronic inflammation within interstitial spaces, the thrombin- Par-1 receptor attachment persists and FAK reversal is not inclined to occur.

When capillary cell outer membrane immune trafficking is hijacked by chronic inflammation, immune arsenal entrance into the interstitial spaces, which includes un-vetted clotting factors, will result in unanticipated clotting-thrombosis events that compromise the involved end organ. The persistent presence of thrombin on capillary cell outer membranes helps to stage this likelihood.

Free Radicals: A Team that can Block or Fuel Inflammation

Free radicals are a diverse group and can result from lifestyle generated *vascular inflammatory free radicals* or can be the result of cellular combustion in the form of mitochondrial exhaust. This type of free radical is known as an *ROS (reactive oxygen species)* and can take the form of *superoxide* (along with hydrogen peroxide) in the case of mitochondrial energy combustion or as *hydroxynitriles* (cousins to cyanide) in the case of nitric oxide combustion. Both superoxide and hydroxynitrile exhaust can work for the cell in the form of beneficial feedback loops to outer membranes and other organelles, as long as one type of combustion is not excessive. When combustion swings back and forth, free radicals are effectively neutralized by antioxidants and actually participate in inflammatory breach removal. When combustion does not swing, free radical exhaust accumulates, antioxidants get depleted and damage to membrane surfaces and DNA results.

Free radicals can also be generated by the metabolism of interstitial space disease venues that include cancer and bacterial cells. As they multiply and grow in mass within the interstitial space they will release their own toxic exhaust. Regardless of where they come from the accumulation and lingering of free radicals will eventually doom the intestinal space and end organ.

The accumulation of capillary cell mitochondrial free radical exhaust (ROS) generated from persistent energy combustion can play a pivotal role in expanding immune arsenal trafficking into interstitial spaces. Not only does superoxide or hydrogen peroxide attach to outer membrane surfaces to initiate activation of protein kinase switches and reduce cAMP, but they can also crosslink naked mitochondrial and nuclear DNA. This has the devastating effect of silencing protein synthesis thereby slashing outer membrane receptor replacement and sharply cutting into mitochondrial volumes within the cell. Capillary cell outer membranes pseudocapillarize, which severely impacts choreograph, and enables more rebel immune arsenal entrance into the interstitial space. As the disabled capillary cell is compromised from signaling effective feedback loops to its allies, their outer membranes become hijacked pawns to chronic inflammation, rogue immune arsenal and disease venues.

When it comes to mitochondrial free radical exhaust in any human cell, *balanced energy and nitric oxide combustion* becomes critical to offsetting excessive free radical exhaust buildup. In the case of capillary and endothelial cells, a balanced swinging of mitochondrial combustion between energy and nitric oxide enables capillary cells to regenerate infrastructure while also switching purpose within the interstitial space and end organ. As important, cycling combustion enables antioxidants to replenish.

A balanced capillary cell mitochondrial combustion is best accomplished by reducing or blocking the other two sources of free radicals. Those include vascular inflammatory free radicals, largely occurring as the result of lifestyle choices, and preventing the development of free radical inducing disease venues, like cancer, fibrous scarring or infections.

One pathway ROS utilizes to increase trafficking of immune arsenal into interstitial spaces is through the outer membrane *xanthine-xanthine oxidase complex*. When ROS activate this complex, the adenylate cyclase-6 conversion of ATP to cAMP is blocked thereby decreasing cAMP levels. This will then cascade activation of certain protein kinase switches to pathway increases in immune arsenal trafficking into the interstitial space. Like the thrombin- Par-1 receptor, if this free radical driven xanthine-xanthine oxidase remains activated, mitochondrial combustion stays in energy mode, makes more superoxide free radical exhaust to thereby push declines in free radical generated damage to DNA. Immune arsenal entrance into the interstitial space becomes more random, rebel and offensive to the integrity of the end organ.

Abundant and persistent free radical interference into the internal affairs of the endothelial and capillary cell will never produce good outcomes to the interstitial space or end organ. It is best to keep free radicals to a minimum and well diversified so that antioxidants can eliminate them. The best sequence to limit free radical interference is to minimize vascular inflammatory free radicals, decrease the risk for chronic disease venues, and keep the capillary cell dance in full pivot and swing.

Bradykinin: Inflammatory Expansion on Steroids

Bradykinin is another molecule that can rapidly expand inflammation, if often connected to allergic responses, and is activated with the release of histamine from mast and basophil cells. Circulating bradykinin originates from the precursor *kallikrein* which is produced in the liver. When kallikrein is activated to bradykinin, it becomes a powerful vasodilator, causing endothelial cell smooth muscles to relax. This can have an immediate and sometimes dramatic reduction in blood pressure to at times cause *circulatory or anaphylactic shock*. In these instances, blood pressures can drop so low that they cannot support vital organ function. As blood pressures fall, bradykinin increases endothelial and capillary cell outer membrane permeability to trafficked immune arsenal into interstitial spaces of affected end organs. The capillary cell outer membrane permeability mechanics of the bradykinin pivot likely involve reducing cAMP, activation protein kinase switches, followed by activation of Rhoa-ROCK-FAK and then CAM exposures.

Bradykinin (and histamine) activation often occurs as a result of an inhaled particulate (allergen), bee sting, snake bite or injection/ingestion of a drug. The release of bradykinin can have very serious consequences from loss of consciousness from low blood pressure to dizziness, shortness s of breath, chest pains, wheezing (bronchial asthma), angioedema (dangerous diffuse swelling of the skin, mucous membranes, throat and tongue), as well as hypoxia and ischemia from reduced blood oxygen concentrations. In some instances, involving chronic inflammation and disease venues, bradykinin can be part of a chronic inflammatory response from chronic exposures to a drug, particulate, infectious agent or cancer.

Bradykinin activation co- partners with histamine release from mast and basophil cells and the activation of IgE immunoglobulin. The trio becomes additive to the substantial release of immune arsenal into the interstitial spaces of sinus tracts, mucus membranes, pharynx, nose, throat, lungs or intestinal tract. Signs and symptoms can range from mildly irritating to life threatening.

The antidote to bradykinin is circulating *angiotensin converting enzyme (ACE)*, or angiotensin II, which is activated by feedback loop signals involving the liver, lung and kidney. When angiotensin II is activated, it reverses arterial vessel smooth muscle relaxation. Blood pressures are thereby restored and hypoxic-ischemic risks to end organs reduced. As this occurs, dizziness and consciousness improves as blood flow to the brain improves.

Chronic inflammation can hijack bradykinin to perpetuate disease venues. As bradykinin is activated, more rebel immune arsenal and edema fluid enters the interstitial space, thereby providing an optimal medium for blocking the capillary cell dance, and increasing risks for infection, scarring and cancer growth. As this occurs, nose, sinuses, lungs and to some extent intestines are continuously harassed by allergic type symptoms that include sneezing, post nasal drip, cough and wheezing, skin rashes, nausea, abdominal cramping and diarrhea. Besides reducing all vascular inflammatory free radical exposures, additional lifestyle adjustments that include a strict avoidance of bradykinin and histamine triggers become mandatory. These include avoidance of specific allergens, particulates, toxins, and in some cases gluten and lactose.

Histamine-The Prototypical Inflammatory Expander

Histamine expands interstitial space inflammation commonly in the intestines, sinuses, nose and lungs. Depending on the health of the capillary cell dance will determine whether histamine is helping or hurting the interstitial space. Histamine is found in high concentrations in *mast cells, circulating basophils and platelets.* When signaled by feedback loops that likely involve a mesenchymal cell response to a particulate, toxin or allergen, mast cells or basophils within the interstitial space bind to endothelial and capillary cell histamine (H1) receptors and release histamine granules. The released granules goose capillary outer membrane permeability to trafficked immune arsenal. Included in the goosing is the release by mitochondria of calcium ions and energy. If the offending particulate or allergen is removed, all is good. If not, the smoldering allergen effect makes the capillary cell outer membranes vulnerable to permanent histamine release.

Associated with the merging of calcium ions and ATP on capillary and endothelial cell outer membranes, are the repeating patterns involving the turning on of protein kinase switches, the blocking of adenylate cyclase-6 and the activation of Rhoa-ROCK-FAK-and CAM receptors. The histamine response is most common within interstitial spaces in the sinuses, nose, lungs and intestinal tract. Its release is often accompanied by the release of IgE from eosinophils and the activation of kallikreins to bradykinin.

With chronic interstitial space inflammation, histamine release can become detrimental and spiral increases into the interstitial space of additional and unnecessary immune arsenal. This penetration of rebel immune arsenal will smokescreen efforts to remove real threats to the interstitial space while providing momentum to block the capillary cell dance. The proinflammatory chain reaction provides impetus for the induction by rebel immune arsenal of an alternative feedback loop signaling system, and hijacking capillary cell outer membranes with these rogue signals. This results in an allergen-histamine induced proinflammatory chain reaction that disables the capillary cell, subverts the interstitial space immune arsenal and mesenchymal cell network and diminishes the end organ while punctuating any combination of itchy eyes, post nasal drip, rhinorrhea, sneezing, cough, nausea and diarrhea.

Eventually the chronic inflammatory momentum provides impetus for scar tissue (lung and sinus scarring), recurrent and chronic infections (sinusitis, rhinitis, bronchitis, enteritis), autoimmune diseases and even cancer growth. All of these outcomes promulgate chronic fatigue and different types of pain that include headaches, chest and abdominal pains, and in some instances, generalized achiness. At this stage of disease escalation, a bonanza is created for the medical industrial complex to intervene with tests, and treatments which placate but don't address root causes of chronic inflammation.

When Growth Factors Go Rogue

Vascular endothelial growth factor, also known as *VEGF*, is produced in different types of cells including immune arsenal, endothelial and capillary cells. Based on what cell and when in the inflammatory cycle VEGF appears, it will have different effects on interstitial space inflammatory cascades. Factor in whether the capillary cell or chronic inflammation controls inflammatory cascades and the presence of VEGF within interstitial spaces or attached to capillary cell membranes could be beneficial or menacing to inflammatory breach elimination.

When capillary cells produce VEGF as part of its choreography to eliminate inflammatory breach, it often nuances renewal or refurbishment of the interstitial space. It typically involves endothelial and capillary cell division, for the construction of new vessels, to improve oxygen delivery to the end organ, which may be compromised from chronic inflammatory residuals. Ineffective oxygen delivery could be as a result of compromised blood flow from obstructive plaque downstream larger blood vessels or from scar tissue or other inflammatory residuals within the interstitial spaces of capillary and end organ cells.

When capillaries are dancing, properly reading cues from the interstitial space and properly choreographing, they produce VEGF which then binds to outer membrane receptors to activate protein synthesis and replication of cells. The presence of VEGF on outer membranes in these conditions would imply that inflammatory breach within the interstitial space has been contained or eliminated, capillary cells are dancing, and mitochondria have impetus to swing combustion to nitric oxide. The goal would be to respond to end organ demands for more nutrient and oxygen. Creating new blood vasculature to increase blood volumes, and hence oxygen and nutrient delivery, would address this concern.

The paradox of capillary cell VEGF production is that it may not work if downstream arteries are incapable of delivering more blood flow due to their own basement membrane problems. In this setting, provided the downstream larger arterial vessels cannot free up more blood flow from collateral arteries, no amount of VEGF induced capillary cell replication will satisfy end organ demands. When this occurs in heavily oxygen dependent end organs like heart, brain or retina, end organ cells have only one choice, to atrophy, reduce function or die. Heart failure, macular degeneration and dementia result.

Capillary cell VEGF production is designed to resuscitate an ailing interstitial space and end organ. Selected benefits of capillary cell VEGF production include:
- Increases capillary cell *outer membrane-vesicle fusion* to accommodate movement of energy driven large-bulky molecular transport (albumin, immunoglobulins).
- Increases *VVOs* (clustering of transport vesicles and vacuoles at the outer membrane) for *reverse* transport (exocytosis) of large molecules from capillary cell cytoplasm back to blood plasma.
- Initiate cell division (including protein synthesis and mitosis) and migration of capillary and endothelial cells to form new blood vessels.

VEGF production can be beneficial in conditions where there is interstitial space recovery from free vascular free radical impingement, chronic inflammatory disease venues or blunt trauma. In these scenarios, endothelial and capillary cell VEGF production is controlled by capillary cell feedback loops. In this setting VEGF attaches to capillary cell outer membranes to activate *MAPF (mitogen activated protein kinase)* switch, which then sparks initiation of *angiogenesis*. The growth of new blood vessels will assist in wound healing and end organ recovery.

In chronic inflammatory conditions, where rogue immune arsenal has the feedback loop upper hand in the interstitial space, VEGF production can by capillary cells becomes misguided and may even be parlayed to advance disease venues that include cancer growth or infectious spread. In this venue, VEGF production can cascade malignant chain reactions of other growth factors such as *PDGF (platelet derived growth factor)* and *TGF (transforming growth factor)*. When released for the wrong reasons these growth factors only help perpetuate interstitial space cancer growth or infectious spread. In fact, as capillary cells replicate for the wrong reasons, what additional oxygen delivery they do provide to the interstitial space may be diverted and used by cancer cells or infectious agents to grow and metastasize.

What becomes clear, is how rebel immune arsenal within interstitial spaces can use feedback loop signals that induce growth factor production for the benefit of chronic inflammatory disease venues. This is more likely to occur when the capillary cell itself becomes disabled from a blocked dance and excessive mitochondrial energy combustion. When capillary cells are in control of interstitial space choreography, VEGF and growth inducers can be beneficial to interstitial space and end organ recovery. The opposite occurs when rogue influences control the interstitial space and have hijacked control of capillary cell outer membranes.

Deficiencies in VEGF, TGF and PDGF can be just as damaging to the interstitial space. In this scenario, capillary cells, either loss of nuclear DNA, outer membrane receptors or mitochondrial volumes cannot produce enough growth factors to facilitate their own refurbishment or cell division which in effect compromises and ages the capillary cell. When they can't replicate, replace or refurbish their infrastructure based on interstitial space or end organ demands for oxygen and nutrient, end organ cells atrophy or die commensurate to how compromised capillary cells have become.

In summary capillary and endothelial cell production of VEGF, and the families of other inducible growth factors, participate in an intricate feedback loop signaling system that involves capillary cell response to interstitial space and end organ demands that is linked to interstitial space sanitation and end organ function. When growth factor release are in the control of chronic inflammation, cancer growth and infectious spread are more likely outcomes to the interstitial space and are accompanied by atrophy and death of end organ cells. Growth factors going rogue is an invitation for rapid expansion of the end organ end game.

TNF-Tumor Necrosis Factor: A Cluster Bomb that Resolves or Expands Inflammatory Breach

Tumor necrosis factor (TNF) is a powerful cytokine which like VEGF, can be released by a variety of different cells to mosaic a beneficial response to inflammatory breach. TNF plays a significant part of macrophage and monocyte response to inflammatory breach elimination. It does so through attracting clusters of additional cytokines towards the breach, which prepares the offender for phagocytosis (swallowing) by monocytes or macrophages. Just like with VEGF, when TNF is properly choreographed by capillary cells, the response plays out to breach removal, a return of optimal interstitial space sanitation, the pivot and swing of capillary cell outer membranes and mitochondria which is then parlayed to capillary and mesenchymal cell regeneration and improved end organ function. When TNF is under rogue influences, TNF release supports a much different agenda that supports rather than eliminates inflammatory breach.

One ways in which TNF clusters cytokine trafficking into interstitial spaces is through by the *albumin-vagabond effect*. When interstitial space inflammation incites a surge of albumin into the interstitial space, it can carry with it a powerful cache of proinflammatory momentum that includes attached cytokines, and the potential to shift fluid and electrolytes into the interstitial space by affecting hydrostatic and oncotic pressure gradients across membrane surfaces. With interstitial space inflammatory breach, monocytes and macrophages release TNF, which among other things induces albumin to enter the interstitial space. As it is actively transported into the interstitial space across capillary cell outer membranes, it not only carries a cytokine payload, but also effects *hydrostatic and oncotic pressure gradients* across membrane surfaces. The net effect is to force edema fluid into the interstitial space, causing the capillary cell to become dehydrated relative to the interstitial space. As capillary cells become dehydrated, their outer membranes increase permeability to additional immune arsenal trafficking.

With chronic interstitial space inflammation, TNF production can go rogue to induce non-sequenced proinflammatory immune arsenal cascades that involving liver production of *CRP (C reactive protein)*, interstitial space clustering of misguided cytokines, mistake prone macrophage *phagocytosis,* and inappropriate CAM exposures resulting in wayward neutrophil and lymphocyte attachments. Any or all of these misfires will expand ineffective inflammatory responses to inflammatory breach. With capillary cell in control of chorography TNF release will assist in processes that eliminate inflammatory breach.In chronic inflammation it will do the opposite.

As chronic inflammation induced TNF is produced, capillary cells stop dancing and their outer membranes become prone to hijacking by rogue immune arsenal feedback loop signals. The bias includes decreases in cAMP, protein kinase on switches, voltage gradients, and inappropriate activation of CAM receptors. Gap junction orifices stay open and channels widen as gap junction infrastructure loses capacity to pace immune arsenal entry into the interstitial space. In addition, because of edema fluid, gas exchange to the end organ is compromised predisposing to hypoxia and ischemic injury. This hypoxic interference can cascade production of capillary cell VEGF and growth factors.

With chronic interstitial space inflammation, TNF release by monocytes and macrophages results in sloppy, uneven and inappropriate release of cytokines and growth factors that cascade a cluster bomb of immune mistakes within the interstitial space. This results in acceleration of chronic inflammatory anti-organ disease venues that can quickly compromise the end organ as cancer growth, infectious disease expansion and hypoxic- ischemic events surge. Regardless of how chronic inflammation exploits TNF, it gateways a disabled capillary cell and blocked capillary cell dance, pseudocapillarization of its outer membranes and sharp reductions in mitochondrial volumes. In most instances, inappropriate TNF surges within the interstitial space are fueled by abundant vascular inflammatory free racial fuel.

Prostaglandins: Rejuvenation or Accelerated Senescence

The prostaglandins family of inflammatory mediators offers another example of how a family of molecules can work for or against the interstitial space depending on the controlling influence. With ideal capillary cell choreography, the prostaglandins group mosaics a diversified mix of different effects that facilitate inflammatory breach containment and elimination. Said differently, when choreographed correctly, prostaglandin release from different cells will provide beneficial feedback loops that enables elimination of an inflammatory breach. If prostaglandin production is not choreographed by capillary cells a darker feedback loop signaling system will not only block inflammatory breach removal but enable propagation of interstitial space disease venues.

All nucleated cells within the human body make prostaglandins. Depending on the inflammatory signal (see the corresponding figure below), *arachidonic acid* (a fatty acid also known as arachidonate in the figure below) is converted by *cyclooxygenase enzymes (also known as COX 1 or 2)* to form *prostacyclin 1 and 2.* Conversion to prostacyclin in capillaries induces smooth muscle relaxation in downstream arterioles to widen their lumens and increase blood flow to upstream capillary beds. Prostacyclin production in capillary cells commonly occurs when interstitial space inflammatory breach has been eliminated and mitochondrial nitric oxide combustion has been initiated. Within the interstitial space, white blood cells will convert arachidonic acid to *leukotrienes,* which generally bias increases to inflammatory expansion. In platelets, arachidonic acid is converted to *thromboxanes,* which activate platelet adhesion to induce clotting and thrombosis. Thus prostaglandin production in capillaries, white blood cells and platelets can be either pro or anti-inflammatory. This complex mix makes capillary cell choreography critical to the successful management of interstitial space sanitation and end organ function.

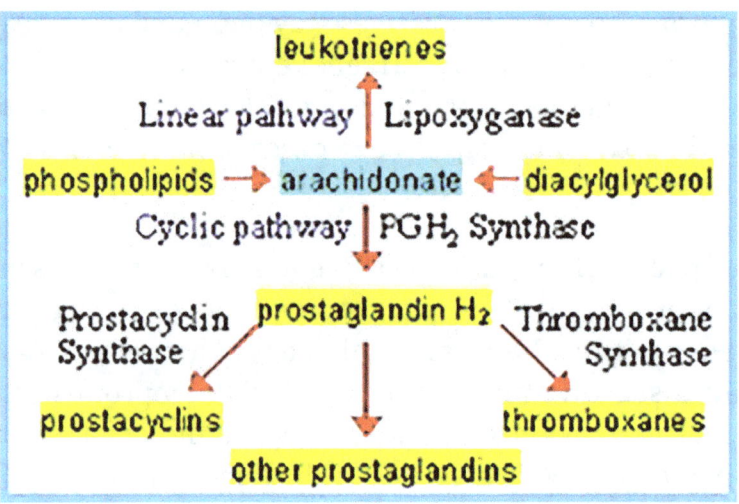

The complex mosaic of prostaglandin synthesis is demonstrated by how capillary and endothelial cell prostacyclin production effects platelet production of thromboxanes. When capillaries produce prostacyclin, it feeds back to platelets within their interstitial space domain to blocks thromboxane synthesis, which blocks platelet aggregation and thrombosis. Capillary cell prostacyclin production thereby biases reductions in immune arsenal trafficking, as it increases blood flow to the end organ.

As part of the anti-inflammatory cascade, capillary prostacyclin increases endothelial cell *PPARs (peroxisome proliferator activated receptor)* while facilitating white blood cell production of in*terleukin(IL-10),* while also inhibiting white blood and mesenchymal cell production of interleukins (IL-1,6) and growth factors. These adjustments help finalize inflammatory breach mop-up while biasing the swing of mitochondrial combustion to nitric oxide. The inflammatory stakes run high If capillary cell PPARs activation and white blood cell IL-10 induction does not occur. In this scenario, with sustained capillary cell prostyclin inhibition, there is overproduction of white blood cell leukotriennes and platelet thromboxanes resulting in escalation of a chronic proinflammatory momentum.

The following table summarizes how endothelia prostacyclin production is critical to counterbalancing proinflammatory cascades.

	Prostacyclin effect	Mechanism	Cellular response
Classical functions	Vessel tone-decrease blood pressure	$\uparrow$cAMP, $\downarrow$ $\downarrow$membrane Ca^{2+},	$\downarrow$Smooth muscle cell contraction $\uparrow$Vasodilation
	Anti-proliferative-block scarring	$\uparrow$cAMP $\uparrow$PPAR	$\downarrow$Fibroblast growth
	Antithrombotic-block clotting	$\downarrow$Thromboxane-A2 $\downarrow$PDGF	$\downarrow$Platelet aggregation $\downarrow$Platelet adherence to vessel wall
Novel functions	Anti-inflammatory-	$\downarrow$IL-1, IL-6 $\uparrow$IL-10	$\downarrow$Proinflammatory cytokines $\uparrow$Anti-inflammatory cytokines
	Anti-mitogenic	$\downarrow$VEGF $\downarrow$TGF-β	$\downarrow$new blood vessel growth $\uparrow$endothelial cell membrane remodeling-Increase receptor density

In summary, endothelial and capillary cell prostacyclin production is signaled when conditions within the interstitial space favor successful removal of inflammatory breach. The likelihood of this occurring improves when the interstitial space vascular inflammatory free radical fuel is substantially decreased. Doing so enables endothelial and capillary cells to produce prostacyclin, which overrides cascading proinflammatory biases that involve prostaglandin synthesis in white blood cell and platelets. Lifestyle adjustments, particularly related to a plant based diet and regular exercise, become powerful tool s that help keep the capillary cell dance robust. Doing so not only causes capillary cells to rejuvenate, but also the powerful feedback loops that healthy capillary cells generate, will pace and stem removal of interstitial space inflammatory breach, rejuvenate either directly or reciprocally mesenchymal and end organ cells, and optimize end organ function. To the extent that capillary cells are enabled to dance is to the extent that chronic inflammation is countered, and with it, the competing rogue feedback loops that it conjures.

Leukotrienes: Cytokines that Frame Choreography

Leukotrienes are families of different cytokines that are produced by white blood cells that mosaic inflammatory expansion or contraction. Depending on whether endothelia or chronic inflammation is in control of interstitial space sanitation will determine whether leukotriene cytokines erroneously expand or contract inflammation. It is the robust capillary cell dance and the choreography that it conjures that largely determines the effectiveness of a leukotriene response to an inflammatory breach. Because of how important leukotriene messages are to signaling of capillary cell outer membranes, if they come from rebel white blood cells to create a disruptive or confused message, the capillary cell outer membranes lose their rhythm to eventually enable a chronic inflammatory coupe to the interstitial space. Capillary cell outer membrane hijacking gets easier when vascular inflammatory free radicals are continuously harassing endothelial and capillary cell basement membranes.

A key intermediate in the production of leukotrienes within white blood cells is the fatty acid -arachidonic acid (arachidonate). In the presence of activated lipoxygenase enzymes, arachidonic acid is converted into leukotriene cytokines.

With inflammatory breach to an interstitial space, white blood cells are choreographed into the interstitial space, which includes their released leukotrienes. They act as messengers to other interstitial space white blood and mesenchymal cells, but are particularly important to capillary and endothelial cell outer membranes, as they facilitate the next steps of choreography in the breach containment and elimination process.

The initial breach assault team of early immune responders, include cytokines (IL-6), neutrophils and platelets. As neutrophils attach, roll, enter the gap junction channel, and emerge into the interstitial space, they are converting arachidonic acid to leukotrienes B4 (LTB4), C4(LTC4) and D4(LTD4). When released, these leukotrienes signal back to endothelial and capillary cell outer membranes to sequence next step choreography from the blood plasma. The early responder leukotriene release potentially cascades:

- Expand capillary cell outer membrane trafficking of either more neutrophils or inducer-helper T lymphocytes, depending on how breach confinement is progressing.
- Effect blood flow dynamics to the capillary cell bed.
- Stimulate T cell lymphocyte (inducer and/or helper T cells) migration from the blood or lymph tissues.
- Aggregate specific immunoglobulins along with complement and platelets for purposes of interstitial space mobilization.
- Help to direct albumen entrance into the interstitial space along with its cytokine payload.
- Nuance production and integration of additional cytokine inflammatory expanders or contractors from capillary and mesenchymal cells.
- Cause the potential release of growth factors (TNF, TGF -transforming growth factor, VEGF-endothelial cell growth factor, PDGF -platelet derived growth factor, as well as integrating other immune arsenal into the mix, which include histamine, thrombin and bradykinin, among others.

After elimination of inflammatory breach, inflammatory breach mop- up becomes the critical next step in downshifting capillary cell outer membrane permeability which then swings mitochondrial combustion to nitric oxide. This step, assures future quality assurance to interstitial space sanitation, as capillary cell "replace, repair and replicate" what is worn out while stemming and pacing similar effects to its interstitial space allies.

What are the mechanics of capillary cell outer membranes that permit a permeability downshift? It comes down to membrane *COX II, omega three fatty acids and the production of HEPE.* When signaled from interstitial space leukotrienes, capillary cell outer membranes switch their *COX II* enzyme substrate *from* arachidonic acid to *omega three fatty acids, such as EPA.* By utilizing omega three fatty acids instead of arachidonic acid, outer membrane COX II enzymes produce HEPE (hydroxyeicosatetraenoic acid) which facilitates activation of adenylate cyclase-6 to increase cAMP, while also blunting activation of several protein kinase switches.

HEPE gets released into the interstitial space and forms a feedback loop with white blood cells. It signals neutrophil lipoxygenase enzymes to switch leukotriene production to *lipoxins (LX, LXA4, LXB4).* Lipoxins trigger inflammatory breach mop-up operations by signaling monocytes and macrophages to engulf inflammatory debris. Lipoxins also cross talk with platelets to block thromboxane production, which blocks thrombosis. In addition, lipoxins work within the neutrophil framework to induce production of *resolvins,* which cascade additional mop- up operations. Thus the switch of capillary cell COX II production from arachidonic acid (omega 6) to omega 3 fatty acids (EPA) to produce HEPE triggers cascades of mop-up feedback loops that reduces the interstitial space inflammatory response and downshifts capillary cell outer membrane permeability to trafficked immune arsenal.

Specifically, the HEPE induced production of neutrophil lipoxins and resolvins cascades:

- Increasing interstitial space monocyte and macrophage phagocytosis.
- Reduced capillary cell CAM receptor exposures
- The likelihood of gap junction orifice closure.
- The push of capillary cell outer membrane reconfiguration from oval to flat
- Inhibits the release and effects of growth factors (VEGF, TNF, PDGF, TGF), histamine, and thrombin among others.

S1P: The Leukotriene that Facilitates Mop-up Operations

Like HEPE, *S1P (sphingosine)* can also facilitate downshifts in immune arsenal trafficking by affecting endothelial and capillary cell outer membrane permeability. Sphingosine is produced in white blood cells and platelets, and cascades feedback loop momentum in synergy with lipoxins and resolvins.Sphingosine binds to interstitial space albumin which then will attach to capillary cell outer membrane receptors known as *EDG 1,3,5, and 8.* Activation of EDG reduces capillary cell outer membrane permeability to immune arsenal trafficking by presumably increasing membrane cAMP and shutting down protein kinase switches. This cascades to reduce CAM receptor exposures. Binding different EDG receptors can result in reducing permeability to different inflammatory mediators. For example, binding to one EDG receptor could blunt VEGF. Binding to a different EDG receptor could facilitate closure of the gap junction orifice and so on. Thus S1P turns albumin into a facilitator of reduced capillary and endothelial cell permeability. In this sense, albumin can work membrane permeability in both directions depending on what is bound to its receptors.

If chronic inflammation is in control of the interstitial space, white blood cells and platelets are never signaled to produce S1P. Even if for some reason it did get produced its effects would be disabled by how disabled the capillary cell had become and the subsequent effects of outer membrane pseudocapillarization. In this scenario S1P-albumin binding either does not occur or becomes unrecognizable to feeble capillary cell outer membrane EDG receptors, as they are either atrophied or are silenced by ineffective replacement.

When EDG 1 is bound by the S1P- albumin complex, a proposed reduction in capillary cell outer membrane permeability to immune arsenal may be as follows.

- In combination with lipoxins and resolvins among others, S1P-albumin complex binds to EDG receptors to initiate increased adenylate cyclase 6 activity to increase cAMP and turn off protein kinase switches.
- This biases capillary cell outer membrane cascades that favor calcium ion and ATP retrieval back to the mitochondrial matrix.
- This pushes capillary outer membrane counter activation of FAK, certain G proteins, and PPARs to sway membrane infrastructure to reduce CAM exposures, close the gap junction orifice and reduce vesicle and transcellular transport into the interstitial space.
- The surge in calcium and ATP back to mitochondria produces a powerful feedback loop to swing combustion to nitric oxide. As interstitial space breach is eliminated, interstitial space sanitation is restored and capillary cells quality assurance is maintained.
- There is considerable proinflammatory backlash to these feedback loops with abundant vascular inflammatory free radical fuel, a blocked capillary cell dance and the inability of capillary cells to lead the feedback loop signaling assault on interstitial space inflammatory breach.

Ang-1: A Fly in the Chronic Inflammatory Ointment

Angiopoietin one or Ang-1, is another and different kind of growth factor that counterbalances capillary cell outer membrane trafficking of immune arsenal. Angiopoietin 1 is part of a family of four or more angiopoietins that are produced by mesenchymal cells. They can bind to capillary cell outer membrane receptors, effect tyrosine kinase switches and bias reductions of immune arsenal trafficking into the interstitial space. As such Ang-1 helps protect the capillary cell pivot and swing dance and the mitochondrial swing of combustion to nitric oxide. The counterpart to Ang-1 is Ang-2, which has the opposite effect on tyrosine kinase, immune arsenal trafficking, and outer membrane capillary cell permeability.

With the emergence of chronic inflammatory influences within the interstitial space, mesenchymal cell production of Ang-1 decreases and Ang-2 increases. This reversal creates the potential for more proinflammatory momentum and the likelihood of unregulated and non- sequenced immune arsenal entrance into the interstitial space thereby perpetuating chronic inflammatory purposes.

When Ang-1 attaches to capillary cell outer membranes to effect tyrosine kinase, the activated switch blocks calcium ions from effecting the transmembrane sodium and potassium pump. This causes accumulation of calcium ions within the capillary cell's cytoplasm and the potential for increasing membrane voltage gradients and membrane cAMP. This in turn cascades reductions in outer membrane permeability and trafficking of immune arsenal and CAM receptors become unexposed. In this sense Ang-1 could work in conjunction with FAK, HEPE, lipoxins, resolvins and sphingosine-1.

What is clear is that capillary outer membrane permeability to trafficked immune arsenal can get messed up when their choreography is disrupted. In this case, chronic inflammation can increase Ang-2, which then chain reacts capillary cell outer membrane targets that block its dance and promote the cell's decline.

Herein lays the medical industrial treatment paradox. By treating disease venues while ignoring chronic inflammation, the ladder still has a leg up on interstitial space control. This means that one disease venue, within a given interstitial space and end organ, can get replaced with another one based on what kind of disease venue opening is created by the different treatment interventions. Without reducing chronic inflammatory fuel, disease venue treatments will be short lived and predispose to additional disease venues mimicking a vicious cycle.

The discoveries of how feedback loops can drive the activation of FAK, HEPE, lipoxins, resolvins, S1P and angiopoietin-1 to reduce capillary cell outer membrane permeability to trafficked immune arsenal thereby enabling the capillary cell dance, provides insight into how important the elimination of interstitial space inflammatory breach is to optimizing interstitial space and end organ homeostasis. Chronic inflammation, through the use of rebel white blood cell interstitial space signals can influence mesenchymal cells to increase Ang-2 production while also cascading disruptions that effect HEPE, lipoxins, resolvins, and S1P to name just a few. The capillary cell dance gets blocked, and the interstitial space bushwhacked. So much of this horror will hinge on how well the endothelial and capillary cell can protect their own basement membranes and interstitial space hygiene from free radical impingement.

Intestinal Microbiome: One Equivalent of Immune Stem Cells

Are bacterial populations within the intestinal lumen really a key component to our immune arsenal? Accumulating evidence suggests that interstitial space inflammation within our end organs is directly influenced by what we eat. And what we eat has a direct influence on what are *intestinal microbiome* looks like. With a diet high in sugar and processed foods, the optimal intestinal microbiome is decimated and replaced by opportunistic bacteria that reduce absorption of quality nutrient (*leaky gut*) and favor absorption of toxins, sugar and partially digested food. This reversal dramatically pushes a systemic proinflammatory agenda that begins with the microbiome, extends to endothelia, cascades to involve liver and fat cell metabolism and is soon followed by proinflammatory cycles involving multiple end organ interstitial spaces.

In this broad sense, this cascade that starts with the intestinal microbiome makes bacteria a kind of stem cell to immune function. A diet heavy in plant fiber, or say cruciferous vegetables, selects an optimal microbiome which reduces leaky gut, enhances immune function and is anti-inflammatory. Diets high in sugars, trans-fats, processed foods, salt and nitrosamines (red meat) do the opposite. Excess sugar consumption does so much wrong in so many ways. Not only does is gateway addiction to more sugar ingestion and possible exposures to other drugs, alcohol and toxins, but it increases circulating vascular inflammatory free radicals (AGEs, LDL cholesterol, non HDL cholesterol, triglycerides, lipo(a), and homocysteine). The sugar rush to the liver will cause liver cells to transition to become more like fat cells (fatty liver transformation) and to increase fat cell influence on all metabolism.

Besides sugar and highly processed foods (snack foods, processed grains and certain dairy products) the microbiome can be aggravated by poor water sanitation, malnutrition, intestinal worms, parasites and antibiotics.

The ramifications of a leaky gut deserve more attention. Not only is it associated with a disrupted microbiome but it can be considered a form of chronic inflammation that begins within intestinal crypts, spreads to involve the interstitial spaces of portal vein endothelia, to eventually involve liver sinusoids and their endothelia, interstitial spaces and hepatocytes. As liver manufacturing and distribution are disrupted, the toxic influences spill over into the central circulation, where it then effects the rest of the vascular tree and end organs they serve. The net effect of this proinflammatory assault being spewed into the central circulation is to increase interstitial space inflammation throughout the body, disable the capillary cell dance and perpetrate chronic inflammatory disease venues in multiple locations. It becomes only a matter of time before brain fog, depression, allergies and asthma, recurrent infections, heart disease and painful arthritis ensue. Different types of end organ scarring, cancer growth and autoimmune diseases are not far behind.

With advanced age, and in some cases inherited predispositions, *gluten and lactose* intolerances can further impact the microbiome. This usually means that with aging, diets must be even more stringent when it comes to refined carbohydrates, dairy products and grains. If possible diets should be plant based, whole food and accented by beans, herbs, water, green tea, coffee and small amounts of dark chocolate. Chronic interstitial space inflammation begins with our diet and how it affects the microbiome. Learn to say no to the morning donut, bacon and sugared coffee or just about anything that is prepackaged.

Chronic Inflammation: The Toxic Stew that Stirs the Interstitial Space Pot

Preventing chronic inflammation within interstitial spaces of end organs enables the capillary cells to dance. This optimizes interstitial space homeostasis, improves end organ function and promotes wellness. The anti-inflammatory lifestyle adjustments affect the entire vasculature and all end organs. As such lifestyle becomes the lifeblood to wellness and the foundation to holistic health. Preventing chronic inflammation minimizes replacement of capillary cell signaling influences from the darker feedback loops generated from rebel immune arsenal. Traditional medicine diagnosis and treatment is based on disease venues, which are late and more difficult to treat manifestations of chronic inflammation. At this end stage, not only does treatment get risky and side effect prone, but it often cascades other disease venues. Treatment paradigms involving disease venues are increasingly becoming more like a Rubik's cube.

Not that disease treatment models are not well intentioned, but because they come so late in the chronic inflammatory scheme, they are risky. That is, they are more likely to fail, cause treatment complications, can be very expensive and often create more treatments as complications and other diseases escalate. This is why so many of our elderly or those with compounding chronic illnesses get pushed into an assembly line of tests, procedures, treatments and doctor appointments. They are being cycled within the medical industrial complex, as Pavlovian dogs and food reinforcement. The only comfort they feel comes from the hope of the next test or treatment. This imprisonment within disease treatment is a terrible way to live and will eventually break the medical bank.

Taking a fresh look at chronic inflammation at an earlier stage, *before disease venues have occurred*, only makes practical sense. So far the momentum of disease treatment is too far entrenched to affect meaningful change. Making the necessary adjustment by tackling chronic inflammation early and head on nips its root cause, prevents disease rather than treating it, and limits the fatigue, chronic pain and aging fall-out that inevitably occurs.

Implied in this discussion is that interstitial space cytokines, white blood cells, immunoglobulins, complement and mesenchymal cells can expand or contract inflammation to cause disease or prevent it based on whether capillary cells or rebel white blood cells are in control of the interstitial space. Implied is whether messages received by capillary cell outer membranes from the interstitial space are working towards inflammatory breach removal or against it. In the case of rebel immune arsenal, the feedback loop signals create a rogue message to capillary cell outer membrane receptors and switches that creates enough disarray that chain reacts additional mistakes of immune arsenal entry into the interstitial space, thereby creating a new chronic inflammatory entity within the interstitial space. This inflammatory matrix (Graph 3, appendix) matures as its alternative feedback loop system hijacks control of capillary cell outer membranes, while also causing capillary mitochondria to get stuck in energy combustion. The superoxide free radical exhaust, and the sticking of energy combustion that it causes, becomes a lethal knife to mitochondrial and nuclear DNA. As the capillary cell declines from silenced DNA, the interstitial space becomes the sole property of chronic inflammation and the emergence of disease venues from the chronic inflammatory anti-organ. Instead of white blood and mesenchymal cells, immunoglobulins, albumin, complement and platelets eliminating inflammatory breach and sanitizing the interstitial space, the reverse happens. The feedback loops created by rebel white blood cells and misguided cytokines they release scramble intent to perpetuate interstitial space anarchy.

Adding advanced age into the mix doubles down on chronic inflammatory risk from the accumulation of DNA cross linkage over time. The silencing of protein synthesis that occurs as a result of this cross linkage, limits repair, replacement and, replication of outer membrane receptors and mitochondrial volumes, even in the presence of pristine interstitial space hygiene. This means that with aging, reducing the vascular inflammatory free radical fuel must be even more stringent. It also means that for a given volume of fuel, the attendant risk to the interstitial space and capillary cell escalates with age. One cigarettes smokes at age 65 is like 3 smoked at 25. The same hold true for donuts, alcohol, other drugs, lack of sleep, stress or inactivity. Cheating at 65 creates a 3x risk for inflammatory momentum compared to age 25. Disease venues will populate interstitial spaces faster and with more virulence.

With the emergence of disease venues, the end organ becomes set up to fail. Capillary cells have stopped dancing, have lost feedback loop control of the interstitial space as the outer membranes have been hijacked. The membrane receptors have pseudocapillarized and their mitochondrial volumes have shrunk. Everything is now in place for a chronic inflammatory interstitial space coupe. The disabled capillary cell becomes a conduit to what the chronic inflammatory anti-organ requires. As scarring, cancer, infections and thrombosis increase, the end organ becomes increasingly dysfunctional. Pain and fatigue partner with accelerated aging and the chronic inflammatory circle is complete. Death becomes a forgone conclusion as all organ systems misfire in harmony.

CHAPTER 12

TRAFFICKING METHODS

When capillary cells elicit a robust dance, the interstitial space rhythm is in sync. The implication is that the capillary cell is facilitating the right mix of immune arsenal to keep interstitial space hygiene optimal. It also implies that vascular inflammatory free radical fuel within interstitial spaces is kept at manageable levels. In addition to capillary cell outer membrane trafficking mechanics that involve cAMP, protein kinase switches, CAM receptors and voltage gradients, immune arsenal trafficking is also affected by d*iffusion, facilitated diffusion and, active transport.*

When capillary cells are dancing, they have ushered into the interstitial space a precise and sequenced immune arsenal network, that subsequently signals back to capillary cell outer membranes, a correct cadre and cadence of next step immune arsenal arrivals to eliminate interstitial space inflammatory breach. The elimination enables capillary cells to downshift outer membrane permeability and swing mitochondrial combustion to nitric oxide creating regeneration. The dance cycle can thereby repeat itself into perpetuity. Chronic inflammation within interstitial spaces never gets established, and the pacing of rejuvenation by capillary cells to its mesenchymal and end organ cell allies, ensures a quality longevity without pain or fatigue. Part of this built in quality assurance that stems from the capillary cell dance is how its outer membranes utilize diffusion, facilitated diffusion and active transport to express interstitial space hygiene and optimize end organ function.

Passive Transport: Providing the End Organ it's Life-Blood

Passive transport across membrane surfaces is most commonly facilitated by diffusion, which is how most gases move across membranes. In this instance, gases will typically follow concentration gradients, where they move through membrane surfaces based on which side of the membrane has less concentration of the gas. This movement does not require energy or adjustment of membrane voltage gradients, receptor switches. The movement across membrane surfaces of oxygen, carbon dioxide, other gases and nitric oxide follow this diffusion pattern. Since oxygen is essential for all end organs to function, based on mitochondrial combustion, the diffusion of this gas across capillary membrane surfaces into the interstitial space is mandatory for their effective function. One combustion bi -product of oxygen utilization is carbon dioxide. It too must be capable of diffusing out of the end organ cell, into the interstitial space and through the capillary cell to enter the central circulation via the red blood cell, where it is carried to the lung alveolus and dropped off as oxygen is picked up. This cycling of oxygen and carbon gas exchange is accomplished by diffusion across multiple membrane surfaces.

Diffusion across membrane surfaces is typically blocked by chronic inflammation within interstitial spaces. It can occur as a result of reductions in blood flow to the capillary bed, the accumulation of edema fluid within the interstitial space, or the buildup of scar tissue, cancer growth or infectious spread. In these cases, oxygen delivery and carbon dioxide release is diverted, subverted, blocked, or utilized by other cells for other purposes. When this occurs, the end organ cannot function well because it does not get enough oxygen. Over time this causes end organ cell can atrophy or even death. Diffusion of oxygen and carbon dioxide is most effective when the interstitial space is not encumbered by chronic inflammation influences or disease venues.

Diffusion of gases is not only effected by chronic inflammation's disease venues, but also from the effects of endothelial and capillary cell pseudocapillarization. As basement membranes thicken it impedes the pace of gas diffusion. When coupled with downstream obstructive plaque, and disease venues, end organ oxygen deficit accelerates and their decline is more rapid.

Chronic interstitial space inflammation has also biased capillary cell outer membrane configuration to stay oval rather than flat. The oval configuration means there is less surface area exposure between capillary basement membrane and end organ outer membranes making gas exchange between them more difficult. The more perpetually oval the capillary cell becomes, the less capacity it has to nurture the end organ.

In optimal homeostasis between capillary and end organ cells, gases freely move across membrane surfaces from higher to lower concentrations. *Equilibrium of gas tension* occurs when the concentration of the gas on both sides of the membrane is the same. This is best accomplished when the gas crossing the diffusing membrane is unencumbered with inflammatory residues. Optimizing gas equilibrium between membrane surfaces tension is critically important in oxygen sensitive end organs such as brain, retina and heart.

The passive diffusion of gases across membrane surfaces becomes an important feedback loop to the capillary cell dance and the swinging of capillary cell mitochondrial combustion. For oxygen to diffuse freely, vascular inflammatory free radial fuel should be minimized, interstitial space inflammatory breaches eliminated and the capillary cell made as flat as possible. The shadowing of the interstitial space with scar tissue, immune complexes, blocked blood flow, chronic or recurrent infections and cancer cells, makes diffusion complicated and ineffective. In these settings the end organ goes from first to last in the diffusion food chain.

Facilitated Diffusion and How Endothelial Outer Membranes Gate

In contrast to gas exchange between membranes, the movement of electrolytes (sodium, potassium, chloride, bicarbonate, among others) across membrane surface is accomplished by *facilitated diffusion*. Electrolytes are ubiquitous to all membrane surfaces and participate in surface membrane exchanges to facilitate voltage gradients. They may be positively or negatively charged and include potassium, sodium, chloride, bicarbonate and phosphate. Within capillary cell outer membranes, electrolytes seek equilibrium by penetrating *slits* and *diaphragms* that can be specific for each electrolyte. The positively charged sodium and potassium could fit through one slit or diaphragm whose membrane surface is negatively charged, whereas the negatively charged chloride, bicarbonate and phosphate, would move through slits and diaphragms that carry a weak positive charge. Outer membrane slits and diaphragms enable electrolyte facilitated diffusion across membrane surfaces without utilizing energy for active transport. With chronic inflammation, outer membrane slits and diaphragms diminish thereby decreasing facilitated diffusion of electrolytes and biasing reductions in outer membrane voltage gradients. This becomes another trademark of capillary cell outer membrane pseudocapillarization.

Another example of facilitated diffusion across membrane surfaces involves *solubility*. Molecules with more fatty acid exposures are known as *lipid or fat soluble*. Since membrane surfaces are predominantly composed of lipoproteins, molecules that have more lipid or fat within their structure will cross membrane surfaces more readily on the basis of their solubility. On the other hand, if the traversing molecule is more *water soluble*, it will meet resistance when attempting to traverse through the membrane. Since many molecules, particularly complex ones which have both water and lipid solubility, there movement through the membrane becomes more complicated and is based on the preponderance of lipid and water solubility and the permeability characteristics of the membrane. In other words, a water soluble molecule will have a better chance of pushing through a capillary cell outer membrane when its permeability or trafficking of immune arsenal into the interstitial space has increased. Thus chronic inflammation within interstitial spaces tends to break down outer membrane solubility enabling a more diverse group of molecules to penetrate through them and into the interstitial space. This often does not bode well for effective capillary cell choreography of breach elimination.

Fat soluble vascular inflammatory free radicals, such as small particle LDL cholesterol, triglycerides, non HDL cholesterol and lipo (a) will use their fat solubility to cross endothelial membrane surfaces to gain entrance into the interstitial space where they can attach and inflame basement membranes. In this manner, proinflammatory free radicals molecules can act in stealth as they seamlessly move through endothelial and capillary cell membrane surfaces.

Besides solubility, slits and diaphragms, another example of facilitated diffusion involves endothelial cell outer membrane *pores*. Pores come in different sizes thereby enabling different sized molecules passage through them. Within a given pore, are diaphragms and slits, which carry weak positive or negative charges similar to those not in pores. My utilizing slit and diaphragms within a givens pore, outer membranes have capability of mobilizing different sized molecules through membrane surfaces without the need for energy. In this manner, a *positively charged* diaphragm membrane within a pore can attach to a *negatively charged* transport protein to facilitate mobilization across the pore membrane or visa- versa. Once attached the carrier protein can either be moved through the pore membrane utilizing a vesicle or transport channel or the attached molecule can be released from the protein carrier, migrate through the slit or diaphragm, and into the endothelial cell's cytoplasm. The utilization of pores, slits and diaphragms enables specific transport proteins entrance into the pore often with a specific payload drop-off. With chronic inflammation and pseudocapillarzation of capillary cell membrane surfaces, pore diversity decreases. When pores become a one size fits all, this substantially limits the capacity of different sized protein carriers access to slit and diaphragm attachments within a given pore. This limits effective capillary cell choreography in the management of interstitial space inflammatory breach and becomes one more nail in the capillary cell coffin.

The use of an outer membrane positive or negative charge to receive a molecular attachment in a different sized pore is known as a *gate. Endothelia and capillary cell pore diversity, and the slits and diaphragms they harbor,* gate trafficking of immune arsenal into and out of the interstitial space. As such they become key pieces to capillary and endothelial cell choreography. This arm does not require energy, but works in conjunction with diffusion of gases and energy driven activation of protein kinase switches, the rotation of CAMs the opening of the gap junction orifice and the active transport of different immune arsenal through the capillary cell via the gap junction, vesicles and transport channels.

When gating does not involve pores, it becomes a tool of adjusting endothelial and capillary cell outer membrane voltage gradients. When outer membrane gating breaks down from chronic inflammatory influences within the interstitial space, membrane voltage gradients decrease enabling increased permeability trafficking of mistake prone immune arsenal. When capillary and endothelial cell outer membrane gating is optimal, the membrane acts like a "catch and carry" as it utilizes voltage gradients pores, slits, diaphragms, lipid solubility and different protein carriers and their payload specific passage across the membrane. This has the opposite effect of pseudocapillarization, as it affords the best method of sanitizing the interstitial space through sequenced choreography of specific immune arsenal. Passage into and out of the interstitial space becomes well-intentioned and purposed.

Facilitated diffusion can also occur on the basis of outer membranes *ligands,* or *second messenger receptors.* As an example, an incoming negatively charged molecule binds to a membrane positively charged molecule in a slit or diaphragm. This attachment not only enables transmigration of the molecule or electrolyte through the slit or diaphragm but can also feature a ligand binding. When the attachment becomes a ligand it becomes a chain reacting signal that activates other membrane mechanics, such as protein kinase switches. Activation of these switches then may nuance different CAM exposures. Facilitated diffusion, through a variety of outer membrane operational mechanics, can optimize endothelial cell outer membrane homeostasis to facilitate interstitial space sanitation and end organ function without utilizing oxygen and energy.

Active Transport: When all Else Fails, Energy Provides a Way

Active transport across endothelial and capillary membrane surfaces provides the fit and finish to immune arsenal trafficking into and out of interstitial spaces. If diffusion and facilitated diffusion set the table for trafficking, energy driven active transport provides the necessary tools for many of the the final steps of immune arsenal mobilization. Active transport usually requires the membrane budding fo vesicles and transport channels for carrying large bulky molecules or cells through the endothelial or capillary cell in processes known as *endocytosis* (from blood plasma to interstitial space) or *exocytosis* (interstitial space to blood plasma).

Active transport is required when larger molecules or cells are pushed against an *electric, mechanical, osmotic or hydrostatic membrane gradient*. Without energy to facilitate working around these barriers, these molecules will have no other way of passing across the membrane. The budding of capillary and endothelial outer membrane vesicles is a common method employed to transfer bulky proteins, such as albumen or immunoglobulins, but can also involve other proteins or white blood cells. Transcellular transport utilizing newly created channels through the cytoplasm is another method of mobilizing large and bulky molecules. To facilitate vesicle and transcellular transport outer membranes require quick infusions of energy (and calcium ions) to membrane surfaces. This is derived from mitochondrial combustion of energy.

Mitochondrial energy is released as triphosphorylated molecules ATP or GTP with ATP being attached to magnesium and transported to the outer membrane surface. Together with released calcium ions, in addition to the construction of transport channels and vesicle budding, calcium ions will affect the contraction of actin-myosin fibrils, membrane voltage gradients, the reduction of membrane cAMP and activation of protein kinase switches. All of this chain reacts increases in capillary cell outer membrane permeability while prepping the outer membrane and gap junction for increased immune arsenal trafficking through it.

In some cases, manipulating capillary cell outer membrane voltage gradients require the use of energy to increase or decrease permeability. In these instances, energy is required to push calcium ions against concentration gradients. This calcium push that enables a higher concentrations of calcium ions in the capillary cell's cytoplasm is known as *antiport*-active transport. This lowers the outer membrane voltage gradient which then chain reacts facilitated diffusion of smaller lipid soluble cytokines to slip through the membrane.

When inflammatory breach within interstitial paces is near completion, capillary cell outer membranes are signaled by neutrophils, lymphocytes and mesenchymal cells to *de-escalate* inflammatory mediator movement into the interstitial space. Feedback loop mechanics are put into place within capillary cell outer membranes that increase cAMP, turn off protein kinase switches to inactivate CAM receptors. As capillary cell outer membrane permeability decreases, gap junction orifices and channels narrow, and transcellular transport channels and vesicles deactivate. ATP and calcium ions accumulate in the capillary cell cytoplasm and feedback to mitochondria to swing combustion to nitric oxide. The switch in mitochondrial combustion to nitric oxide pivots capillary cell purpose from protecting the interstitial space to preserving its quality assurance and optimizing end organ function.

Conclusions

The sequenced dispersal of any molecule by capillary cells to and from the blood and interstitial spaces of end organs requires interactive combinations of outer membrane diffusion, facilitated diffusion and active transport. In aggregate they serve as check and balance signals to endothelial and capillary cell outer membranes which are designed to affect immune arsenal trafficking and interstitial space sanitation, or alternatively, to goose end organ function. As they do this they enable the capillary cell dance thereby providing necessary shifts in outer membrane permeability and mitochondrial combustion. This provides impetus for capillary cell rejuvenation and becomes a marker to the cell's future quality assurance. The dance provides powerful pacing feedback loops throughout the interstitial space that enable its allied partners similar regenerative benefits. Molecular impingement on capillary outer membranes involves a continuous compilation of nuanced effects that increase or decrease momentum for exposures of different protein kinase switches, CAMs, pores, slits, diaphragms, and voltage gradients which then lead to blocking or enabling energy driven vesicle and transcellular channel transport. If this delicate symbiosis is hijacked by chronic inflammation, the intricate feedback loop choreography created by the enormous capacity of capillary cell outer membranes to assimilate and respond to signals is lost.

When molecular impingement on capillary outer membranes is occurring in the context of a robust capillary cell dance, they facilitate a signaling system that feeds back to mitochondria, combustion, nucleus, and other organelles to make intracellular adjustments. In addition, endothelia send signaling feedback to interstitial space allies, the end organ, adjacent capillary cells, downstream endothelium and distant end organs. This signaling input engineers interstitial space sanitation while optimizing end organ function. As this occurs, the robust capillary cell dance is facilitating necessary quality assurance of its infrastructure via repair and replacement of worn out proteins while pacing a similar venue to its allies.

All of this balance and counterbalance provided by capillary cell choreography becomes vulnerable to attack from chronic inflammatory influences within the interstitial space. It becomes predictable when the interstitial space and capillary-endothelial cell basement membranes are impinged by vascular inflammatory free radicals. Eventually this impingement implodes capillary cell function by disrupting enough of their infrastructure to cascade a blocked capillary cell dance, the sticking of mitochondrial energy combustion, superoxide toxicity, nuclear chromosomal decay, and the subsequent loss of mitochondrial volumes and pseudocapillarization of outer membranes. Feedback loop ownership of the interstitial space gets transferred to chronic inflammation. Welcome, disease venues, the demise of the end organ, and waves of pain and fatigue.

CHAPTER 13

PARODIES TO INFLAMMATORY MEDIATOR TRAFFICKING

Chronic end organ interstitial space inflammation plus genetic aberrations, either inherited or acquired will tsunami proinflammatory momentum. It is clear that endothelial and capillary cell disaster begins with vascular inflammatory free radical impingement into interstitial spaces, expands to include our own immune arsenal and then utilizes both to decay the capillary cell, block its feedback loops signals and initiate disease venues which eventually destroy the end organ. The capillary cell seizing up of mitochondrial combustion in energy mode triggers the capillary cell decay as superoxide free radicals accumulate, crosslink and silence nuclear and mitochondrial DNA. As coded protein replacement is silenced, aging outer membrane receptors, infrastructure components and mitochondrial proteins are not removed and quality assurance within the capillary cell dissipates. The capillary cell slide is exactly the opening that chronic inflammation desires to expand operations.

As chronic inflammation garnishes interstitial space favor, capillary cells whither to become functional illiterates. As capillary cells lose their signaling influence the feedback loop pieces are picked up by the increased interstitial space presence of rebel immune arsenal. As feedback loop momentum changes hands, the march towards converting mesenchymal cells to the alternative path is well under way. When capillary cell outer membranes have been successfully hijacked and mesenchymal cell allegiance completed, the chronic inflammatory fix is in. With the introduction of the anti-organ, the disease venue game plan has been established.

This becomes the third and late stage of chronic inflammation and forms the basis for diagnosis and treatment in modern allopathic medicine. Cancers, scar tissue, infections, autoimmune complexes or thrombosis all couple in different combinations the make the end organ's interstitial space a mosaic of destruction. As the end organ ship sinks, fatigue and pain compound its failure.

Disease treatment can inflict disruption to the chronic inflammatory game plan, but this becomes only temporary unless the underlying mechanics of chronic inflammation are equally addressed. This means a robust reduction in vascular inflammatory free radical fuel and a return of the capillary cell dance. Lifestyle choices become medicine and when used comprehensively, become the antidote to vascular inflammatory free radical fuel. If reduced substantially it can jumpstart the capillary cell dance. Doing so, frees up capillary cell mitochondria to swing combustion to nitric oxide, which keys rejuvenation and the rebirth of feedback loop control of the interstitial space. This becomes the linchpin to unraveling chronic interstitial space inflammation.

Can optimal lifestyle adjustments complemented with age appropriate supplements and as needed medicines actually refresh the endothelial and capillary cell dance? The answer is an unqualified yes, but not indefinitely as acquired nuclear chromosomal aberrations will silence protein replacement and limit how much capillary cells can rejuvenate. As their quality assurance evaporates, so does their capacity to exert feedback loop control of the interstitial space. Could stem cell rejuvenation be the answer to increasing nuclear DNA senescence? A tantalizing thought of life eternal but lifestyle fundamental s must still remain in place for any intervention to have long term impact.

The relationship of capillary cells to their partners can be summarized in parodies. As parodies go, anti-inflammatory lifestyles induce *good manners* to endothelial and capillary cells in the following ways:

- By practicing personal hygiene through the pivot and swing dance. This enables the ultimate hygiene for capillary cells nitric oxide induced combustion supports refurbishment of outer membrane receptors, mitochondrial volumes, and infrastructure.
- Maintain intimacy with their life partner, the end organ.
- Attempting to always stay in touch with best friends (mesenchymal cells).
- Making sure to track and pay close attention to messages from interstitial space white blood cells and platelets.
- To always check times, places and references when receiving signaling messages from cytokines, or immunoglobulins.
- To listen and communicate with colleagues (adjacent endothelial and capillary cells).
- To stay in touch with downstream distant relatives (from large vessel endothelia to capillary cells from distant end organs).
- To never forget the importance of communicating with in-laws (communication with other end organs).
- To adapt to sudden changes in prevailing conditions. This could involve sudden swings in end organ oxygen and nutrient demands or a response to a surge of interstitial space free radicals or other menace.
- When making executive decisions about trafficking into the interstitial space to be aware of the big picture.
- To be a good citizen and stay informed of new developments occurring elsewhere. This includes within its immediate domain, downstream, or to other end organs.

Endothelial-Capillary Cell Hygiene = Interstitial Space Hygiene = Optimal End Organ Function

For capillary cells optimal hygiene is linked to interstitial space sanitation. For the interstitial space, the limitation of vascular inflammatory free radical fuel and the penetration of disease venues becomes the parody equivalent of regular teeth brushing, the Mediterranean diet, getting 7 hours of continuous sleep, exercising regularly and avoiding undue stress. In the case of the capillary cell these practices enable optimal rhythm of their pivot and swing dance. When the dance is robust interstitial space sanitation is fine tuned. This means that capillary cell mitochondria are counterbalancing their combustion as outer membranes are pivoting their trafficking permeability.

Maintaining capillary cell hygiene directly correlates to lifestyle. In practical terms it means:

- Sharply reducing simple sugars and trans-fat intake, to treat exercise as a daily habit, to reduce weight to a BMI (basal metabolic index) of 25, to eliminate smoking, alcohol and drug addictions, and to reduce through all means possible small particle LDL cholesterol, triglycerides, non HDL cholesterol, lipo(a), homocysteine, elevated blood sugars and blood pressures. Insomnia, sleep deprivation and obstructive sleep apnea should be addressed and prevailing behaviors that are inducing stress need modification.
- Optimize anti-oxidant, mineral and vitamin levels that are biased to decrease with age. Doing so improves infrastructure performance and reduces risks for lingering toxic free radical exhaust.

Good capillary cell hygiene boils down to optimal lifestyle choices. It does not require fancy gadgets, expensive drugs, gym memberships or other tech gimmicks. It does require taking back control of what your life should *look and feel* like. Your endothelia will say thank you. That thank you ripples to the end organ's they serve.

Always Communicate and Maintain Intimacy with Your Life Partner

The primary purpose of the capillary cell is to serve its lifelong partner, the end organ. To do so it must effectively dance and maintain interstitial space sanitation by removing inflammatory breach. In parody, this translates to keeping the interstitial space house clean. By cleaning the house, its communication and ability to respond effectively to its end organ partner increases several fold. If the interstitial space is not kept clean and becomes preoccupied with free radical debris and disease venues, effective communications with the end organ is blocked. At some point, as disease venues mature, the capillary- end organ cell relationship becomes so strained that they in effect divorce. When this occurs, signaling feedback loop communication is effectively cut off and the end organ stranded.

For effective long term intimacy between the capillary and end organ cell, the capillary cell must *not be distracted* by interstitial space free radical shenanigans. As long as capillary cells can dance their end organ partners should stay happy.

Maintain Communication with Best Friends

Essential for capillary and end organ cell intimacy is the best friend support they receive from interstitial space mesenchymal cells. These close friends maintain surveillance of the interstitial space and frame cytokine responses to identify and remove interstitial space encumbrances that otherwise would impair capillary –end organ cell intimacy. They do this by providing capillary cells with an extra set of *arms, eyes and ears* that address inflammatory encumbrances to the interstitial space platform that may have entered in stealth or were unrecognized at first pass through the capillary cell. Different mesenchymal cell friends carry out different functions within the interstitial space. While some collect intelligence and signal back to capillary cells for immune arsenal reinforcements, others can directly kill-shot intruders. When working in close conjunction with their capillary cell friends, they facilitate a quick reconciliation to inflammatory breach. On the other hand if successfully duped by chronic inflammation and rebel white blood cells, they will betray their capillary cell friends, ignore inflammatory breach, and cause further separation of thee capillary –end organ cell relationship.

Drop Thank You Notes to White Blood Cells and Platelets

Like mesenchymal cells, immune arsenal can make or break interstitial space sanitation. When capillary cells are dancing and feedback loops robust, white blood cells and platelets are choreographed to the interstitial space staging area where they perform their duties in sync to remove inflammatory breach. As they perform, they subsequently release additional signals that enable capillary cells to continue sequencing choreography of trafficked immune arsenal until the breach is removed. Because of their sacrifice capillary cells should send thank you notes to circulating white blood cells and platelets reminding them of their importance should the interstitial space be invaded in the future with a similar breach.

Check References, Dates and Times of Cytokine and Immunoglobulin Messaging

When processing immune arsenal responses, capillary cells must check and cross check intelligence information before committing immune arsenal access to the staging area. These cross checks prevent improperly choreographed immune arsenal entry, which can chain react additional mistakes. The capacity to check and cross check requires a fully functioning capillary cell outer membrane receptor network. Capillary cells must cross check the *context* of the signal to exact a correct response. A growth factor, or other cytokine coming from cell A will have a different implication than coming from a wayward cell B.

Never Forget Colleagues

Fellow capillary cells, particularly those immediately next door, need to work as a team to enhance capillary cell purpose. Capillary cells cannot meaningfully perform their tasks in isolation. Rather capillary cells must come together in aggregate to provide a uniform front. This neighborly relationship requires that they share information through channels known as connexins in their gap junctions.

It also requires that capillary cells remember their colleagues further away. It takes a village of capillary and closely related arterioles to accommodate effective trafficking of immune arsenal into interstitial spaces to eliminate inflammatory breach. In this manner, as capillary cells provide their neighbors with real time intelligence information through connexins, they are also transmitting signals to nearby arterioles to increase or decrease blood flow (oxygen and nutrient) towards them. They do this via nitric oxide gas, endothelin or prostacyclin among others, which act as cytokines to relax or contract arteriole smooth muscle thereby increasing or decreasing blood flow. Capillary cells will also seek collateral assistance from lymphatic and venous endothelia, when additional white blood cell reinforcements are required within the interstitial space or for help in removing interstitial space waste.

Depending on prevailing circumstances within the interstitial space, capillary cells may send signals to far away colleagues for help. These signaling cues require a capillary cell universal language spoken by all endothelia that understands the context of released cytokines. The interpretation helps generate a consensus response from all capillary colleagues throughout the vascular tree. The implication is that capillary cell colleagues, regardless of where they are located, will have the backs of their colleagues, regardless of where they are or what might be going in their own interstitial spaces.

Make sure to Remember Birthdays and Important Events from the In-Laws

The "n-law" distant end organs provide critically important feedback loops to capillary cells by secreting hormones and enzymes that help facilitate capillary cell outer membrane trafficking momentum while improving the capacity of their respective end organs to function. For example, capillary cells, of the blood brain barrier, function optimally when their outer membrane permeability is nuanced by gas, hormone, protein and enzyme input from other end organs, such as the adrenal glands, liver, kidney, heart and lung. The implication is that capillary cell effectiveness is based on the sum of its end organ parts. It behooves capillary cells to remember end organ birthdays, In this manner, it can track how different end organ function may change with age and to make adjustments based on what they are not providing

As an example, all end organ age but in a given individual some may age faster than others based on lifestyle choices. In those who have a 20 year or more history of heavy alcohol consumption, liver cells have often atrophied or have transitioned to become more like fat cells. In these conditions the liver becomes incapable of manufacturing and distributing albumin, clotting factors, complement or certain inflammatory proteins. When this occurs, capillary cells everywhere, including the blood brain barrier, must accommodate for these shortages. The same holds true for the aging kidney and the removal of toxic waste or the scarred up lung and the capacity to execute oxygen and carbon dioxide gas exchange. Each end organ on its own can affect capillary cells, but when their function accelerates downward in aggregate, capillary cells will find it increasingly difficult to accommodate end organ failures.

End organ failures, no matter which disease venue induced them or how advanced they have become, can be stabilized or even reversed if capillary cells are enabled to resume their dance. The dance becomes the signature to healing of the interstitial space and return of end organ function, but can only occur when there is a sharp reduction in vascular inflammatory free radicals. Any other treatment short cuts will be self- limited and doomed to failure.

Ironically, as any end organ fails, the vascular free radical basis for its failure coupled with its lost function will provide proinflammatory momentum to other end organs to fail along with their interstitial spaces. As scarred up lungs reduce oxygen exchange in their alveoli, the deficit ripples throughout the vascular tree to affect all end organs but particularly those that are heavily dependent on oxygen combustion to function, such as heart, brain and retina. The same holds true for a scarred up liver of kidney or an intestine plagued with leaky gut. Capillary cell will adjust to end organ scarring or other disease venues when lifestyle choices reduce vascular inflammatory free radicals, enable their dance, and improve their capacity to respond to interstitial space challenges.

Capillary cell encrypted birthday wishes to distant in-laws and their capillary brethren should be:

- Just remember, when it comes to your interstitial space and vascular inflammatory free radicals, less is better.
- I value your *quid pro- quo.*
- I'll let you know if anything changes on my end and I hope you do the same ASAP.
- I always respect your input into my affairs as you have my back.

I know you are one year older but age is just a number. We are all in this together.

Adapt, Adapt, and then Adapt More

When endothelia are in their youth, they are up to most challenges in the interstitial space. They pivot and swing rigorously in precision with signaling cues that eliminates interstitial space inflammatory breach quickly while adjusting seamlessly to end organ nutrient-oxygen demands. As this occurs, it bolsters its own quality assurance while signaling similar adjustments to its interstitial space allies. Optimal interstitial space homeostasis is a forgone conclusion that in some respects is taken for granted.

The one irreplaceable trait that a robust capillary cell dance accomplishes is its capacity to *multitask.* At any given moment the capillary cell outer membranes may be addressing several different concerns at the same time. When fully equipped, as well as locked and loaded with a full complement of receptors, infrastructure, and mitochondrial volumes, they can manage a variety of simultaneous multitasks seamlessly by adjusting feedback loop signals to their infrastructure, interstitial space allies, end organ and beyond. Effective multitasking enables *adaptivity*. Doing so puts the endothelia in general and the capillary cell in particular in a unique position to master plan the game plan within the interstitial space while also keeping the end organ happy.

Their precise signaling calculus is connected to the vigor of their dance. As capillary cells age this dance is biased to less vigor and this translates to less multitasking and less adaptability. The risks increase for chronic inflammation to man handle the interstitial space. With age, the capacity of capillary cells to dance becomes dependent on sharp limitations in vascular inflammatory free radicals while keeping chronic interstitial space inflammation on a short leash.

When a capillary celli age multitasking is limited by cascading proinfammatory chain reactions that are assisted by chronic interstitial space inflammation. Suffice to say it involves reductions in mitochondrial volumes and pseudocapillarization of outer membranes that are accompanied by ineffective DNA coding for protein synthesis. This translates to capillary cell outer membrane inability to receive and send signals and mitochondria's reduced capacity to provide energy for execution. As their signaling feedback loops wind down and are replaced by those of rogue influences, capillary cells become hijacked bystanders to the agendas of chronic inflammation. This becomes the definition of aging as end organs fail, disease venues mount and fatigue and pain escalate.

Choose Weapons Wisely

Capillary and endothelial cells function as stewards to interstitial space sanitation. That stewardship is at risk when proinflammatory free radical spirals are thrust into the interstitial space. The initial offender(s) are usually vascular inflammatory free radicals. If the fester, seeds are planted for chronic inflammation to find interstitial space footing. To prevent this, endothelial and capillary cells must choose immune arsenal weaponry precisely to eliminate the potential for a chronic inflammatory beach head. Coupled with lifestyle choices that minimize vascular inflammatory exposures to the interstitial space and a recipe is evolved to keep capillary cell dancing and the sanitation of the interstitial space intact.

Sequencing immune arsenal in the management of inflammatory breach is a dynamic exercise in capillary cell choreography as different breaches require a different assemblage of immune arsenal weaponry. The breach scope also requires adjustment in the volume of weaponry used. The success of the weapon response is often dependent on intelligence capillary cells receive in the form of signaling cytokines from white blood cells and mesenchymal cells within the interstitial space. If intelligence has been interfered with (as with chronic inflammation) or misinterpreted, the weaponry brought into the interstitial space will likely be defective. Choosing immune arsenal weapons wisely requires many different moving parts, but ultimately comes down to capillary cell choreography. To the extent that it breaks down is to the extent to which weapons brought into the interstitial space will be used for sinister purposes against the interstitial space, and end organ.

Keep Abreast of Current Events

For capillary cells to effectively dual function as interstitial space gatekeeper and end organ provider, they must be constantly aware of prevailing conditions within their own interstitial space and elsewhere. This not only involves inflammatory breaches and free radical intrusions into interstitial spaces, but also involves making adjustments to sugar or fatty acids that surge in the bloodstream from meal ingestion or collapse from fasting or their utilization when skeletal muscle is being exercised.

With chronic interstitial space inflammation within interstitial spaces, it becomes harder for capillary cells to adapt to prevailing conditions. As might be expected their collective hands are tied in attempting to adjust to proinflammatory momentum within their interstitial space. These attempts often feel uphill and against wind, as they get bombarded with escalating proinflammatory momentum from misguided immune arsenal. Failure can means an end organ interstitial space free fall culminating in a sudden decompensation from a thrombosis (stroke (thrombosis), heart attack (thrombosis)), or sepsis (bacterial or viral streaming into the blood) or fulminant spread of cancer cells.

If capillary cells are dancing they have a better chance of keeping abreast of prevailing conditions. This is because they will be better adept at receiving and sending signals and multitasking. In this mosaic, capillary cells can send measured, intentional and choreographed responses to their interstitial spaces, to protect them while also adapting to whatever is coming at them from the blood plasma. In this sense, capillary cells *protect* and *buffer* their interstitial spaces from untoward blood plasma arrivals.

Parodies: Clarifying the Capillary Cell Village

With emphasis on disease treatment models, the endothelia including capillary cells are often unnoticed as attention is paid to disease outcomes on end organs. While confronting disease head on is and understandable target, it doesn't address how the disease got there in the first place. This lends a blind eye to how chronic inflammation within interstitial spaces takes control to enable disease venues to surface. This means that disease treatment in effect puts the cart before the horse. It ignores how the capillary cell dance is impaired and how that impairment leads to insidious declines in feedback loop control of the interstitial space. Any long term benefit that might occur from disease treatment will be nullified unless the capillary cell can resume its "pivot and swing". Excluding endothelia from the disease treatment master plan will doom the disease treatment master plan.

With endothelial inclusion in the master plan, the importance of their dance is highlighted. In means that vascular inflammatory free radical fuel is minimized. Within the context of capillary cell parodies, it means that all cells involving all end organs and endothelia are interconnected in the management of interstitial space sanitation and different end organ functions. In this manner the capillary cell "social network" ranging from adjacent capillary cells, to those of the interstitial space and beyond, co participate in the management of interstitial space sanitation and end organ function. This defines *holism* and is paced by the capillary cell dance.

It is these feedback loop tie-ins, with their extensive social network, that create the immune mosaic which enters, does its job and then leaves the interstitial space. Leaving the interstitial space sets up the next stage of capillary cell recovery and dispersal of oxygen and nutrient to the end organ. The successful completion of one phase of capillary cell operations creates positive momentum to the next phase, thereby creating a viable life cycle of perpetuating good health starting with the endothelia and capillary cells but also intimately involving the interstitial space and end organ. This capillary cell engagement with its social network village is fast paced, pervasive and perpetual. It expands feedback loop signals as far away as distant end organs but as close as white blood cells within the interstitial space. It involves different waves of cytokines and their signaling attachments to the capillary cell outer membranes and the reverberations that follow. The effective feedback loops management of this diverse array is dependent on how well capillaries are dancing. The more rigorous the dance, the greater the likelihood that inflammatory breach is removed and capillaries can move on and cycle renewal and end organ optimization.

The health of the capillary cell dance is dependent on how much vascular inflammatory free radical fuel is within the interstitial space and how chronic inflammation has utilized this fuel to subvert the immune arsenal to engage into an alternative feedback loop system. The subversion is based on the increasing display of wayward immune arsenal into the interstitial space that are brought in by mistake due to the shutting down of capillary cell outer membrane receptors from pseudoocapillarization. As capillary cell outer membranes pseudocapillarize mitochondrial volumes diminish. The capillary cell specifically and their allied network generally, becomes prone to hijacking and control by a dark feedback loop system engineered by rogue white blood cells that perpetuates disease venues.

When capillaries are dancing, their village communication is dynamic, vascular inflammatory free radical fuel is sparse and chronic inflammation cannot foothold the interstitial space. When they are not, vascular inflammatory free radical fuel is abundant, rebel immune arsenal are more likely to leak into the interstitial space and hijack their membranes and the proinflammatory fires within the interstitial space become increasingly moe difficult to contain. The proinflammatory wave systematically converts mesenchymal cells to the new feedback loop system and leaves no stone unturned as it marches to completely control the interstitial space. Disease venues monopolize entering oxygen, nutrient, white blood cells, cytokines, immunoglobulins, platelets and complement to facilitate their own purpose while leaving the end organ increasingly "high and dry". As this progression continues, the capillary cell becomes a passive conduit, incapable of any meaningful intervention, as long as its outer membrane receptors, mitochondrial volumes and infrastructure are rusting away due to a feeble or nonexistent pivot and swing dance. As chronic inflammation swaps feedback loop control away from the capillary cell the interstitial space becomes a lock for scarring, infections, cancer cells, rogue autoimmune complexes and thrombosis.

CHAPTER 14

HOW TO PREVENT A TRAFFIC TIE-UP

We age and develop chronic illness in proportion to how well our end organs function. This is largely determined by how much sanitation has occurred within their interstitial spaces, which is dependent on how much vascular inflammatory free radical fuel has entered, for how long it has been there, and how it has disrupted the capillary cell dance. When endothelia and capillaries are dancing they perform optimally and trafficking tie-ups don't occur. The interstitial spaces are clean of free radical debris and end organ function waxes in response to capillary cell driven adjustments in blood flow, oxygen and nutrient delivery.

When vascular inflammatory free radical debris accumulates within interstitial spaces, it takes its toll on endothelial and capillary cell basement membranes by attaching, pluming an immune arsenal response, thickening the membrane and making it less amenable to interstitial space signals or end organ requests. It becomes a fundamental ploy of trafficking tie-ups as the emerging feedback loop signaling system of chronic inflammation relentlessly stokes interstitial space momentum.

The emergence of vascular inflammatory free radicals within interstitial spaces usually begins in early adulthood and almost never causes much of a clinical stir, as it does most of its early dirty work in stealth. These free radicals are usually propagated by addictions with some health from weak genetics. They begin with sugar as an initial gateway in pregnancy, but certainly by early childhood through the use of baby food, bread, cereal, and sweets. The addictions through early adulthood may then spread to include drugs, cigarettes and alcohol. These additions increase risks for poor self- esteem, school drop outs, high risk sexual behavior, depression, as well as increases in weight, stress and sleep deprivation. This perfect proinflammatory storm, unless urgently dealt with, will result in a social outlier wrought with psychiatric issues and inability to be meaningfully employed or engage in relationship emotional intimacy. This condition will often spiral into crime, jail, and premature disease venues involving multiple end organs involving infections, cancers, clots autoimmune disorders and premature end organ scarring. Death often occurs decades earlier that peers due to rampant expansion of chronic inflammation and disease venues it creates. In this scenario, capillaries stopped dancing in early adulthood with immune arsenal traffic tie-ups within interstitial spaces spiraling at the same time.

In a sense this pattern is self- repeating and is a reflection of how chronic inflammation operates regardless of what free radical fuel is being used or what genetics are being exploited. If free radical fuel stacks, the capillary cell dance is blocked much earlier and the interstitial space compromised much earlier with trafficking tie-ups and disease venues.

The mechanics of the traffic tie -up are also repeated. Capillry mitochondria get stuck in energy combustion, overheat, produce excessive superoxide exhaust, crosslink and destroy DNA, limit and block effective coding for protein synthesis, thereby negative repair and replacement of outer membrane receptors and mitochondrial infrastructure. As mitochondrial volumes diminish from suicide and outer membranes pseudocapillarize, the capillary cell enables wayward collections of immune arsenal into the interstitial space. The accumulation of unqualified white blood cells into the space becomes a breeding ground for dispersing cytokine signals that further disrupt and confuse capillary and mesenchymal cells. This becomes the calling card for an interstitial space coupe and the hijacking of capillary cell outer membranes by the accumulation of darker feedback loops generated by rebel white blood cells. When mesenchymal cells switch sides, the fix is in and the interstitial space can now be masterminded by the anti-organ.

This interstitial space coupe is the beginning of the end of the end organ. Increasingly isolated from capillary cell support it dives into survival mode, which adjusts its capacity to function into a downward spiral. Within end organs, this usually means atrophy or transition of cells to some other form and the accumulation of scar tissue or amyloid. In the brain, nerve cells atrophy in clumps first in one area such as the prefrontal cortex, but then to involve the entire brain. As brain cells shrink, mesenchymal glial cells secrete amyloid or other forms of scar remnant. As dementia escalates to involve the entire brain, thinking and judgement impairment are also linked to simple reflexes such as walking, balance, hearing and vision. Tremors, falls, stooped gait coupled with poor balance make even getting up from a chair, controlling continence of urine or even swallowing more difficult.

These same events play out in other end organs, but may highlight infections, cancer or thrombosis more than scarring. In the heart, thrombosis or coronary arteries or smaller vessels from plaque buildup is more prevalent and can lead to angina, heart attacks, arrhythmias and heart failure. Shortness of breath may preclude walking even a few feet. Other vital end organs such as the intestines, lung, kidney and liver can develop similar slides in function based on different combinations of scarring, cancer, infections, thrombosis or autoimmune disease. No end organ is immune to the effects of chronic inflammation. The sex organs, gums and skin also will project similar changes. Bones become soft or brittle as tendons, ligaments and skeletal muscle become stiff and prone to atrophy. Peripheral nerves will also atrophy as function is compromised. This chronic inflammatory chain reaction will increase a blend of end organ disease venues, fatigue, pain and accelerated aging.

When it comes to the capillary cell dance, preventing immune arsenal tie-ups and disease prevention within any end organ, who or what controls the interstitial space is everything. If capillaries are in control, vascular free radical volume is marginal, their dance is robust, immune trafficking in and out of the interstitial space efficient, and sanitation effective. If chronic inflammation controls interstitial space dynamics, the capillaries are not dancing, immune trafficking into the space becomes congested, signaling feedback loops become impaired, and inflammatory momentum shifts towards disease venues, fatigue, pain and aging.

I have made a big fuss about the three stages of chronic inflammation (see appendix graph 3). This is to make clear, that chronic inflammation is a process of taking over the interstitial spaces of end organs. It is only at the last stage of chronic inflammation that disease venues manifest. Intervening before disease venues occur by reducing vascular inflammatory free radical fuel while enabling the return of the capillary cell dance only makes sense if taking the long view of wellness and prevention. This also serves notice as a much more pragmatic and cost effective way of administering health care policy. It often takes years if not decades for chronic inflammation to mature to a level to cause disease, yet traditional medicine ignores that maturation process. The later the intervention into the chronic inflammatory process the more difficult it becomes to cure, let alone contain a late disease venue.

The set-up for a chronic inflammatory interstitial space fix within interstitial spaces has three repeating patterns, all of which implode the capillary cell dance, infect their choreography and tie-up effective immune arsenal trafficking. These include:
- *Too much free radical fuel.* Diversification of that fuel creates even more adversity. The ifuel can be a metabolic free radical, such as AGE (advanced glycation end product), LDL cholesterol, lipo(a), homocysteine, or something ingested like alcohol, ingested like an opioid, or inhaled such as a particulate, methamphetamine or some other irritating substance (see the compilation of vascular inflammatory free radicals-Table One, under the section What Confers a Vascular Inflammatory Free Radical).
- Loss of a well-organized immune arsenal response into the interstitial space.
- Loss of effective help from interstitial space mesenchymal cells.

These three patterns are the formula of chronic inflammation and define the first two stages. They build on one another to create proinflammatory momentum that eschews the capacity for capillaries to shift mitochondrial combustion to nitric oxide. Their implosion begins at that point. The evolving *chronic inflammatory dance* within the interstitial space has a much different step to it and utilizes feedback loop chains that have nothing to do with removing free radicals, sanitizing the interstitial space, or supporting the end organ. Rather, these feedback loops signals spread interstitial space trafficking chaos, foster deception, and create opportunity for disease venues. Once capillary cell outer membranes have been fully hijacked by this alternative signaling system, chronic inflammatory control within the interstitial space is established and the space becomes a pick your poison from there. The capillary cell no longer has a sphere of influence except for what is being exploited by chronic inflammation.

By silencing capillary cell outer membrane receptor mechanics, chronic inflammation can signal, through rogue immune arsenal remnants already within the interstitial space, a who's who of reactionary white blood cells, immunoglobulins and platelets that are amenable to just about any purpose. With chronic inflammation in control, that purpose is dark, minimizes the end organ and promotes a heavily biased direction towards disease venues. As immune arsenal tie-ups increase within the interstitial space, and feedback loops jam well intentioned immune arsenal, removal of inflammatory breach becomes a passing memory. In this manner, with the immune arsenal scrambled and the chronic inflammatory fix in, any number of bacteria, viruses, or cancer cells can occupy the interstitial space often accompanied by additional biases towards thrombosis and scar tissue. The burgeoning alternative feedback loop momentum overwhelms well intentioned mesenchymal cells and converts them to darker purposes. The fix is in and the capillary cell is helpless to do anything about it, as long as vascular inflammatory free radical fuel is abundant.

Interstitial space hygiene and efficient end organ function comes down to a gravitational struggle within the interstitial spaces of forces that either favor disintegration or consummation of capillary cell choreography. The stakes are high as untoward outcomes can eventually affect all end organs and interstitial spaces. It is the vascular inflammatory free radical smoldering within interstitial spaces that dials in inflammatory momentum. If capillary cells pivot and swing, we have wellness. If blocked we have fomenting chronic illnesses, fatigue, pain and aging. The interstitial space comes under influence by *who leads*. That leadership is based on lifestyle choices.

Medicines and supplements, while critically important in treating and preventing expansion of disease venues, become meaningless unless we manage good choices involving food, exercise, sleep and stress. Anti-inflammatory strategies, if invoked aggressively and early in the context of disease treatment, should result in substantial reversibility. This means that blood pressure and diabetes can be put in remission and other disease venues, such as cancer, thrombosis or scarring, postponed indefinitely.

Checking in periodically by assessing certain inflammatory benchmarks with a trusted health care provider becomes important in resetting wellness goals. These check-ups should be both instructional and interactive, focused on how to prevent disease, and should make clear connections of disease venue to lifestyle decisions. Besides periodic blood panels, mammograms and colonoscopies, the assessment should always checklist discussions about habits. The goal of the visit is not only to assess symptoms but to understand that symptoms may have origins in our habits.

Nobody wants a life consumed with fatigue and pain yet our lifestyle choices come begging for it. The outcomes to these choices become the equivalent to imprisonment. No one enjoys the entangled process of these medical nightmares that involve countless doctor visits, tests, expensive and dangerous treatments and the side effects that follow. It often becomes a no-win as cancers, infections and clots are strewn across the disease treatment highway and are accompanied by fatigue, pain, dementia, breathlessness and increasing dependency.

If successful, the choice to block chronic inflammatory intent within interstitial spaces will get personal. It involves taking a long view and making tough behavior choices that could nix friendships, a job or even a marriage partner. It involves a deeper understanding about how we find comfort and reward difficult decisions in life. It involves possibly making changes that run contrary to what are genetics are asking for. It requires an understanding of cascading subliminal messages that come from eating sugar, drinking alcohol, using drugs, smoking cigarettes, or getting involved with any other addiction. It will mean taking a fresh look at what is causing our stress or sleep deprivation and making adjustments that could escalate a change in jobs, or relationships. When confronted directly, a sobering understanding will emerge as to why we are not doing well and what we need to do to change it.

Within days and certainly weeks, something good happens. I knew I put that pain and fatigue somewhere but where? And why am I suddenly remembering details? What happened to that AM stiffness and that nocturnal multi trip bathroom experience? Why don't I have a headache and where is all this energy combing from? Come to think of it, I never noticed that wild flower just outside the window before. Those gym shoes are begging for me to put them on and take a walk. Just can't figure out where the pain, fatigue, hangover and headache went. Well, so much for lost baggage.

Robert Buckingham, MD, FACP

GLOSSARY OF TERMS

Abluminal: Endothelial and capillary-cell outer basement membranes that abut the interstitial space and end organ. *Luminal* refers to the endothelial outer membrane glycocalyx that abuts blood plasma.

Acetyl Coenzyme A (acetyl CoA): Is known as the hub of mitochondrial combustion. Both pyruvate (glucose) and fatty acid beta oxidation produces acetyl CoA, which can then be fed into the Krebs cycle to eventually combust energy, or it can be shuffled to ribosomes and the rough endoplasmic reticulum to facilitate protein synthesis or cell replication.

Actin-Myosin Fibrils: Are fibrils attached to the capillary cell continuous outer membrane and infrastructure scaffolding. When these fibrils slide on each other they cause contraction thereby changing the capillary cell configuration from flat to oval or back again. When actin-myosin fibrils slide (contract), they widen the gap junction orifice. This increases trafficking (permeability) of white blood cells or other immune arsenal through the gap junction channel. Actin-myosin sliding is sensitive to the presence of released calcium ions from mitochondria.

Actinin: An infrastructure endothelial and capillary cell outer membrane protein that responds to protein kinase switches and can flex or bend to facilitate exposures of different membrane receptors. This becomes an important cog to capillary cell choreography and how specific immune arsenal are trafficked into the interstitial space. Actinin is one of several infrastructure proteins that service receptor exposure.

Active Transport: The different processes of molecular or cellular transport across cellular membranes that involve the use of energy (ATP). Active transport of immune arsenal across endothelial outer membrane surfaces can occur during inflammatory breach containment or elimination and involves mobilizing different immune constituents in vesicles and transport channels (via exo or endocytosis). Active transport is in contrast to membrane facilitated diffusion or passive diffusion, where energy is not required.

Adenylate Cyclase: An important outer membrane enzyme that stimulates increases in cAMP, which signals a reduction in outer membrane trafficking of immune arsenal into the interstitial space and becomes a strong impetus to a mitochondrial combustion swing to nitric oxide.

Adherens Junction (AJ): Is composed of cadherin adhesion receptors and is part of the gap junction orifice that regulates the pace of immune arsenal trafficking through the gap junction channel. When Endothelial and capillary cell cadherin receptor proteins uncouple to expose their receptors, the gap junction orifice widens to increase the pace of specific white blood cell attachment. Sequenced white blood cells have been rolled towards the orifice by outer membrane selectin receptors.

Adhesion Receptors: The receptors (also known as CAMS or ICAM receptors) are found on endothelial and capillary cell luminal outer membranes and are exposed when triggered by protein kinase switches that facilitate the bending or twisting of infrastructure proteins. Adhesion is accomplished by an exposed receptor attaching a specific white blood cell. The attachment cascades activation of other selectin receptors, which roil the captured white blood cell towards the gap junction orifice, where they are paced within the gap junction channel to eventually get expulsed into the interstitial space staging area.

Adipokines: Inflammatory cytokines secreted from abdominal fat (also known as white adipose). Adipokines becomes a proinflammatory force to increase risk for numerous autoimmune diseases in those with truncal obesity.

Adiponectin: A circulating protein produced by fat cells in response to calorie restriction or regular aerobic exercise. Along with the hormone *leptin* it cascades a reduction in insulin resistance and nurtures desired weight loss. Adiponectin decreases gluconeogenesis, increases triglyceride clearance, upregulates control of outer membrane uncoupling proteins, reduces tumor necrosis factor to favor reductions in endothelial and capillary cell outer membrane trafficking mechanics. It secondarily can reduce vascular inflammatory free radicals such as AGEs, triglycerides and LDL cholesterol.

Advanced Age: Is relative and culture dependent but is defined as being 75 years of age or older. Those with multiple vascular inflammatory risks may appear to be at advanced age at 45, whereas others without any risk factors, may not be considered to be of advanced age at 85.

Advanced Glycation End Products (AGES): Are circulating free radicals in the blood that increase with ingestion of refined sugars or in those with adult diabetes. They do damage by attaching to proteins on membrane surfaces and silence their function while possibly expanding additional inflammation towards their attachment.

Albumen: An important larger protein produced in the liver that can effect membrane pressure gradients, electrolyte and water movement into and out of interstitial spaces, and can attach and carry vagabond molecules for transport across membrane surfaces. As such, the daily production of 15 grams of albumin by the liver is critical to many balancing and counterbalancing mechanics across membrane surfaces, including capillary and endothelial cell outer membranes.

Alpha Helix Bundle Family: A classification of cytokines based on molecular structure and include interleukins 2 and 10 (IL-2,10) and interferons.

Amyloid Deposits: Are secreted primarily from mesenchymal cells within the interstitial space. In the brain, liver, lung, heart and kidney, amyloid is secreted when there is chronic inflammation within the interstitial space. In the brain, the mesenchymal glial cell, which helps compose the blood brain barrier, will secrete beta and tau amyloid and is linked to dementia, tremors, gait disturbance and social isolation. Amyloid can be considered a type of scar tissue and is secreted as hostile conditions within the interstitial space cause end organ atrophy. In the brain, this translates to loss of nerve cell volume with atrophy of dendrites and axons.

Angiogenesis: The process where new blood vessels are produced and is usually induced by released growth factors that cause endothelia to replicate. Like so many released cytokines, this process can be orderly and adaptive to the best interests of the end organ, or if chronic inflammation is in control of the interstitial space, disorderly, and destructive. If angiogenesis is involved in wound healing, it is beneficial. If it is part of a grand scheme of chronic inflammation involving cancer growth, hypoxia from thrombosis or the of spread of infection, it is not.

Angiopoietin 1, also known as ANG-1: Is one of a family of angiopoietins, that can activate receptors on endothelial and capillary cell outer membranes to cause these cells to replicate to form new blood vessels. As discussed with angiogenesis, when this involves wound healing or attempts to increase skeletal or heart muscle tone, it becomes adaptive. Whereas ANG-1 is usually restorative, it is counterbalanced by its cousin angiopoietin 2 (ANG-2). ANG-2 is often increased with chronic interstitial space inflammation and aggravates capillary and endothelial outer membrane capacity to pivot permeability to decrease immune arsenal trafficking into the interstitial space thereby setting up capillary mitochondrial to overheat energy combustion and increase superoxide exhaust.

Angiotensin Converting Enzyme or ACE: Is a circulating enzyme that is regulated by feedback loops through the liver, kidneys and lungs. The enzyme is responsible to the activation of angiotensin II, which is a potent smooth muscle constrictor. By causing smooth muscles of endothelia to constrict, blood pressure increase as lumen diameters decrease.

Antioxidants: Molecules that attach and neutralize free radicals.

Antiport: An effect cellular outer membranes and specifically to endothelial and capillary cells, whereby calcium ions are actively transported (pumped) against their gradient to keep its concentrations much higher within the cell's cytoplasm. This block will bias reductions in outer membrane voltage gradients and permeability to immune arsenal thereby perpetuating additional trafficking.

Arachidonic Acid: An important fatty acid intermediary (considered part of the omega 6 fatty acid family) that is utilized by the enzyme cyclooxygenase (COX II) in many cells, including capillary and endothelial cells, to cascade inflammatory expansion. The utilization of omega three fatty acids by COX II distributes a different intermediary and cascades anti-inflammatory momentum

Astrocytes: A specialized mesenchymal glial cell found within the blood brain barrier complex, that serves as helper cells to the capillary cell in optimizing barrier support. Astrocytes also provide a go between signaling support system for nearby nerve cells and their capillary counterparts. Astrocytes may also malfunction under the guise of chronic inflammation and secret amyloid, which further barriers the relationship between capillary and nerve cell. With brisk reductions in vascular inflammatory free radicals through robust lifestyle adjustments, this amyloid secretion is blocked.

ATP or Adenosine Triphosphate: Is the primary energy unit utilized by capillary and all somatic cells. In capillaries, 90% of basal energy is produced by fermentation within the cytoplasm (without oxygen also known as anaerobic or glycolysis) so as not to diminish oxygen reserve that are required by the end organ. Endothelia including capillary cells only utilize oxygen to make ATP as part of a mitochondrial combustion swing based on signaling feedback loops. The combustion swing is towards energy to support active transport of immune arsenal into the interstitial space to combat inflammatory breach, or nitric oxide, which drives repair and repletion of its infrastructure while increasing oxygen and nutrient to the end organ via increases in blood flow. Energy is released at membrane surfaces when ATP releases phosphorus and degrades to ADP. The concentrations of ATP within the capillary cell cytoplasm serve as an important feedback loop to mitochondrial combustion. If active transport is no longer required at the outer membranes, their levels accumulate and feedback to mitochondria and swing combustion to nitric oxide.

Autoimmune-Complex Disease: This occurs when immunoglobulins misread normal proteins and attach to them as if they are a foreign invader. Their attachment forms an immune complex that chain reacts attachment of complement to signal monocytes or macrophages to attempt engulfing the newly formed immune complex. This has the effect of destroying the membrane, silencing function and chain react adverse sequences that depend on the obliterated protein. This rogue immune complex will get remembered by the immune system to perpetuate additional membrane damage over time. This becomes a disease venue exploited by the chronic inflammatory anti-organ.

Basement Membrane: A capillary cell outer membrane, specific to end organ function, that abuts the interstitial space and end organ cellular outer mem brane. Its morphology blends to the functional requirements of the end organ, as it can function as a filter, sieve or barrier. With chronic inflammation the basement membrane will thicken based on vascular inflammatory free radical attachments and the immune arsenal response towards them. As it thickens, it loses responsiveness to end organ and interstitial space dynamics.

Bifurcating Arteries or Blood Vessels: This is where one artery splits into two arteries. Bifurcations are notorious for developing inflammation, basement membrane thickening and obstructive plaque due to the physics of decreased lumen diameter in the bifurcated vessel and the increase in velocity of blood flow it causes through its lumen. Increased velocity is associated with increased intraluminal pressures and increased shear stress, which can injure endothelial cell outer membranes.

Bradykinin: An inflammatory mediator activated from liver produced circulating kallikrein. Bradykinin profoundly relaxes vascular smooth muscle to decrease blood pressure and biases increases in capillary cell outer membrane permeability of immune arsenal trafficking into interstitial spaces. Bradykinin can cause vascular collapse leading to syncope and loss of consciousness. It is commonly linked to histamine release form mast cells and basophils and as such it associated with allergies, asthma, sinus problems and crampy abdominal pain.

C- Reactive Protein and Highly Sensitive C reactive Protein: Are inflammatory proteins synthesized in the liver that increase in the blood stream with acute and chronic inflammation including chronic inflammatory disease venues. The highly sensitive c- reactive protein, is a more specific inflammatory marker for *vascular inflammation* that is increased with earlier stages of chronic inflammation caused by vascular inflammatory free radicals.

Cachexin also known as Cachectin or Tumor Necrosis Factor (TNF): One of many proinflammatory cytokines that are released to modulate inflammatory expansion. Cachexin can be beneficial or adverse to the interstitial space or end organ depending on what controls the interstitial space (capillary cell or rogue immune arsenal) and from what cell it originates from.

Cadherins Receptors: A family of receptors that are part of the *CAM adhesion network* on the outer membranes of capillary and endothelial cells. This receptor network, that includes selectins and cadherins receptors, facilitate the rolling of white blood cells to and through the gap junction orifice.

CAMs: Is a generic term that encompasses all of the capillary and endothelial cell outer membrane adhesion receptors. CAMS are responsive to kinase activation switches and are exposed by stereotaxic rotation from outer membrane infrastructure proteins.

Capillary Cells: Are a specialized endothelial cell at the very end of the arterial tree that accommodates specific end organ function by primarily modifying their basement membranes to become more like a sieve, filter or barrier. Capillary cells multitask end organ support with interstitial space sanitation while pacing and stemming regeneration of their infrastructure and that of their interstitial space allies.

Catenins: A family of receptors, within the cadherin network, that further nuances white blood cell entry into the gap junction channel.

Cathespin G: An important protease cytokine found in neutrophil granules.

Caveolae: Are small invaginations that are cave like on the capillary cell continuous outer membrane that assist in lipoprotein transfer by forming transport vesicles.

Chain Reactions: In all cells, chain reactions provide *momentum* to increase or decrease function. They can be beneficial or toxic based on what controls the interstitial space.

Chemokines: Are usually very small proteins that function as cytokines. They help mobilize white blood cells within the interstitial space staging area of inflammatory breach.

Chondroitin Sulfate Proteoglycans: An important glycoprotein to capillary and endothelial cell basement membrane infrastructure.

Chronic Inflammation: Any process that festers within the interstitial space of end organs. If allowed to progress through its three stages, it blocks the capillary cell dance, hijacks their outer membranes, dupes mesenchymal cells into switching allegiance and foments disease venues. Chronic inflammation progresses by initiating vascular free radical migration into interstitial spaces, attracting immune arsenal towards them, organizing to form an inflammatory matrix composed of rebel immune arsenal develop a dark and alternative feedback loop system to eventually seize control of the interstitial space to thereby enable the next stage anti-organ to implement disease venues.

Clotting Factors: Are proteins produced in the liver that when activated cascade the formation of a clot or thrombus. They include but are not limited to prothrombin-thrombin (factor II), factor V, factor X, fibrinogen-fibrin.

Collagen: A protein that serves as structural support or glue to membrane infrastructure. In addition to serving important cellular processes, it can also be secreted into interstitial spaces as fibrous scar tissue.

Collagenases: Enzymes that break down collagen. Certain collagenases are used in different wound treatment protocols.

Combustion: Refers to *utilizing oxygen* by mitochondria to manufacture energy or nitric oxide. In contrast to end organ cells, endothelial and capillary cells make 90% of their energy via glycolysis, yet it is their mitochondrial combustion swing that determines success of its dualpurpose as well as quality assurance to future function and that of their interstitial space allies.

Complement : More than 30 different proteins synthesized in the liver and circulating in the bloodstream that compose some of the immune arsenal. When activated they co-participate as part of an immunoglobulin antigen-antibody complex or on the can attach to something foreign without immunoglobulins to disable and prepare the unwanted protein for removal.

Connexins: Membrane proteins that facilitate cross-talk between adjacent capillaries and are known as connexin channels.

Crisscrossing Feedback Loops: Are feedback loops that induce an opposite effect. As an example, when capillaries cell mitochondria combust nitric oxide, they will feedback to end organ cell mitochondria to induce them to combust energy and visa- versa. When capillary cell mitochondria get stuck in energy combustion, their corresponding end organ mitochondria are also stuck in nitric oxide combustion.

Crosstalk: Is the communication between cells that often involves cytokine signals that produce feedback loops. Within interstitial spaces and in the setting of chronic inflammation, crosstalk between capillaries and their allies is scrambled by conflicting signals generated by misplaced white blood cells.

Cyclooxygenase(s)-Are either COX 1 or 2 enzymes that are utilized in different cells to convert either arachidonic acid to prostaglandins or omega 3 fatty acids-EPA/DHA to HEPE in capillary cells. When COX enzymes generate HEPE, there is a cascade favoring anti-inflammatory biases within the interstitial space.

Cyclic Adenine Monophosphate also known as cAMP: Is a critically important messenger of endothelial outer membrane permeability. In the presence of adenylate cyclase, cAMP levels increase in endothelial and capillary cell outer membranes which downshift permeability trafficking of inflammatory mediators into the interstitial space by turning off protein kinase switches. When cAMP levels decrease at the endothelial outer membrane, protein kinase switches are activated, trafficking of immune arsenal through the capillary increases and mitochondria are signaled to swing combustion to nitric oxide. Energy and calcium ions will be released from mitochondria to saturate outer membranes with chain reactions to augment immune arsenal trafficking.

Cysteine Knot: A group of cytokines that are identified by their molecular structure as having a cysteine knot. These cytokines include *transforming growth factors* (TGF) 1-3.

Cytokines: A diverse group of different enzymes/proteins that are released from a variety of cells, including capillary cells, that signal increases or decreases of an inflammatory response. Cytokines often induce chain reactions to amplify their effects. They can be beneficial when choreographed properly by capillary cells or they can be divisive to chain react undesired proinflammatory effects when orchestrated by chronic inflammation. Cytokines can be called different things based on chemical structure, purpose or cell of origin. When released from white blood cells, they are called leukotrienes, or specifically from lymphocytes-lymphokines.

Cytosol: Also known as a cell's cytoplasm.

Diabetes mellitus: Comes in two forms, an autoimmune disease that destroys insulin producing cells in the pancreas (juvenile diabetes or diabetes mellitus type I), or a disease of increasing insulin resistance (adult diabetes or diabetes mellitus type II) that occurs primarily in adults and is linked to genetics, obesity, loss of muscle mass and tone, inactivity and highly processed food. Adult diabetes is defined as a blood hemoglobin A1C level of 6.5 or greater or fasting blood sugar of 126 mg/dl or greater. Prediabetes or insulin resistance is defined as a hemoglobin A1C of 5.7 to 6.4. Diabetes, through the deployment of many different vascular inflammatory free radicals, as well as its effects on cellular gluconeogenesis and preferential fatty acid combustion, increases risk for rapid deployment of chronic inflammation within interstitial spaces.

Diapedesis: The process that describes how migrating white blood cells are brought into or out of the interstitial space staging area through the endothelial-capillary cell gap junction channel.

Dismutase Manganese Superoxide, or Superoxide dismutase or SOD: Are antioxidants that degrade superoxide free radical exhaust but can become deficient with advanced age, malnutrition or if capillary cell mitochondria get stuck in energy combustion. Excessive superoxide ROS can accumulate, degrade DNA and cause coding mistakes leading to the silencing of different synthesized proteins.

DNA: Is harbored in a cell's nucleus or mitochondrial matrix and is stored on chromosomes and protected in the nucleus by a telomere cap. DNA is translated to messenger RNA which is then utilized by ribosomes and rough endoplasmic reticulum to synthesize cellular proteins.

Edema Fluid: Refers to interstitial space edema fluid and is due to the pulling of water from the endothelial and capillary cell into the interstitial space due the effects of albumin. This makes the endothelial cell dehydrated in comparison to the interstitial space and makes it more difficult for the passive diffusion of gas exchange (oxygen and carbon dioxide) between capillary and end organ cells.

Elastase Enzymes: Enzymes that break down certain proteins into smaller constituents.

Elastin: A infrastructure protein that enables membrane flexibility, improving its ability to bend or twist. With aging, elastin becomes less effective in enabling membranes to twist or bend.

Electrolytes: Are considered to be sodium, potassium, chloride, bicarbonate, and phosphate. They are mobilized on different sides of a membrane to create voltage gradients which effect permeability of other molecules moving across the membrane. Electrolyte concentration gradients on different sides of a membrane can occur without the use of energy, such as with facilitated diffusion.

Electromechanical Gradients: Most membranes in all cells have some type of electric-mechanical current running through them. These currents can vary substantially in their strength with the most powerful gradients providing feedback loops that support a barrier function. Membranes that have a strong electric-mechanical gradient are more difficult to penetrate and serve as a blocking membrane against molecular transit.

Endocytosis: An active transport process whereby capillary cell outer membranes bud vesicles or create transport channels to carry different molecular constituents from the blood plasma across the capillary cell and into an end organ's interstitial space. Endocytosis is the opposite of exocytosis. Whereas endocytosis generally expands interstitial space inflammation by adding immune arsenal into the interstitial space, exocytosis contracts that response and is critical to the process of breach mop-up.

Endokines: Cytokines produced by endothelial and capillary cells.

Endoplasmic Reticulum or ER: Can be *smooth or rough*. Rough endoplasmic reticulum contains ribosomes and is a cellular factory for protein synthesis. The smooth endoplasmic reticulum is linked to to mitochondrial metabolism as it becomes an extra storage unit for calcium ions as well as facilitating heme homeostasis.

End Organs: Are the organs that capillary cells respond to that provide a specific function to the human organisms. Examples include the brain, heart, lungs, skin, kidneys, liver, skeletal muscle, intestines, sex organs etc.

Endothelial Cells: Are cells that compose the vascular tree and include large arteries, smaller arteries, arterioles, veins, capillaries, venules and lymphatics. The end organs of all endothelial cells, except capillary cells, are smooth muscle cells. The hygiene of the interstitial space of all endothelial cells is important to how well their respective end organ function.

Entactin also known as Nidogen-1 or NID: Is family of glycoproteins that are integral to capillary and endothelial cell basement membrane structure and function.

Epigenetics: Is the effect that behavior and environmental influences have on our genetics. Proinflammatory behaviors or exposures will significantly impact DNA by enabling an already weak genetic profile to degrade further, or they can induce genetic mutations *denovo* to silence protein synthesis and limit a cell's capacity to signal and respond.

Epithelial Cells: Those cells that are not endothelial cells and are specialized cells that make up all end organs.

Exocytosis: A process that often utilizes energy where a capillary cell extrudes unwanted molecular constituent from its cytoplasm into the blood plasma. Exocytosis is the opposite of endocytosis.

Facilitated diffusion: A process where membranes can have increased concentrations of electrolytes or other molecules on one side of a membrane compared to the other thereby creating a voltage gradient net, without expending energy to do so.

FAD (Flavin Adenine Dinucleotide): Is used primarily in the mitochondrial matrix to receive hydrogen ions from the Krebs cycle or from fatty acid oxidation and donate them back to the cytochromes on the inner membrane for energy combustion.

Fat Soluble: When a molecule is composed primarily of fatty acids it is fat soluble, meaning it can migrate into and across membrane surfaces. Many vascular inflammatory free radicals are fat soluble including small particle LDL, triglycerides, non HDL cholesterol, and lipoprotein(a).

Fenestra: Are pores of varying size, with and without diaphragms. On capillary cell continuous outer membranes, they facilitate choreography of different sized molecules from the blood plasma entering the interstitial space. Generally capillary cell outer membranes that provide a barrier function have fewer fenestra (example-the blood brain or blood retinal barrier).

With pseudocapillarization of capillary cell membranes caused from chronic interstitial space inflammation, the volume and diversity of pores on outer membranes diminish making them less capable of choreography, thereby increasing risk for rebel immune arsenal trafficking through them.

Fibrinogen: One of 13 different clotting factors made in the liver, also known as factor 1. Fibrinogen is converted to fibrin by thrombin, which facilitates the clotting cascade. Fibrin levels decrease in chronic liver disease or when excessive clotting mechanisms are activated such that might occur with cancer, autoimmune disease, bleeding or infections.

Fibroblasts: Part of the interstitial space mesenchymal cell team, that can go rogue if parlayed by enough rebel white blood cell signaling.

Fibronectin: An infrastructure capillary cell outer membrane glycoprotein that can flex to activate integrin adhesion receptors (CAMS) which facilitate attachment of specific white blood cells.

Filamin: An infrastructure capillary cell outer membrane protein that responds to protein kinase switches to flex and then expose different adhesion receptors in similar fashion to filamin.

Foam Cells: Are *macrophage* mesenchymal cells that are laden with fat and are a component of basement membrane thickening and obstructive plaque.

Focal Adhesion Kinase or FAK: An outer membrane protein kinase switch that can nuance membrane infrastructure to increase or decrease different CAM receptor exposures based on what is activating it.

Gap Junction: Is the channel between two adjacent cells. In capillary cells, the gap junction can widen or narrow based on contraction or relaxation of actin-myosin fibrils. The gap junction with its infrastructure becomes a facilitator of capillary cell pace and choreography of white blood cell movement into the interstitial space staging area.

Glial Cells: Form the connective tissue framework within the brain and includes astrocytes. Astrocytes when coupled with capillary and pericyte cells, compose the blood brain barrier. Astrocytes can secrete beta -amyloid and tau both of which act like chronic inflammatory scar tissue, as they intertwine with atrophied nerve cells to block capillary cell engagement.

Glutathione: An all -purpose antioxidant derived from the amino acid cysteine. Glutathione levels decrease with chronic inflammation, advanced age, malabsorption and malnutrition. Along with the antioxidant dismutase superoxide, glutathione helps to degrade the toxic superoxide free radical to carbon dioxide and water.

Gluten: A clump of proteins found in wheat, barley and rye that that can cause an allergic reaction when ingested. Gluten sensitivity may increase with age and includes varying levels of diarrhea, cramping abdominal pain, fatigue and nausea. *Gluten intolerance* is increasingly being recognized as a spectrum of illness that produces varying levels of symptoms that increase with advanced age.

Glycoproteins: Proteins of various sizes and shapes that that have carbohydrate constituents. Glycoproteins can be part of a membrane infrastructure or can function as a receptor. In some instances, glycoproteins can be catabolized and used as energy substrate.

Golgi Apparatus: Is the equivalent of a cell's post office. This organelle processes and final stamps approval for newly manufactured proteins to be utilized throughout the cell. The Golgi apparatus also buds lysosomes from its outer membranes, which can catabolize (break down) a variety of different potentially rtoxic molecules within the cytoplasm.

Helper T Cells: Are white blood cells that are choreographed by capillary cells, based on feedback loop signaling from other white blood and mesenchymal cells into the inflammatory breach staging area to participate in removal of inflammatory breach.

Heme: A tight molecular ring with iron as its centerpiece manufactured in mitochondria with help from smooth endoplasmic reticulum. Heme is used in the cytochrome system to transport electrons.

Heparan Sulfate Proteoglycan Core Protein or HSPG: An important infrastructure protein to capillary and endothelial cell basement membranes.

HEPE: Or hydroxyeicosatetraenoic acid, is produced on capillary and endothelia outer membranes in the presence of COX II enzymes and DHA omega three fatty acid. HEPE causes white blood cells to produce resolvins which signal a downshift in inflammatory expansion, as a mop up operation to inflammatory breach.

HETE also known as Hydroxy- Eicosatetraenoic Acid: A family of at least 7 different enzymes derived from arachidonic acid that facilitates inflammatory expansion within interstitial sapces.

High Density Cholesterol also known as HDL cholesterol: Is the smallest of the lipoprotein particles and is known as good cholesterol. HDL cholesterol is produced in the liver and can vacuum small particle LDL cholesterol from endothelial –capillary cell basement membranes. As such, HDL cholesterol is anti-inflammatory to endothelia.

Histamine: A proinflammatory mediator released by white blood cells (basophils and mast cells). Histamine increases capillary cell outer membrane permeability to a wide range of different inflammatory mediators to expand interstitial space inflammation. Histamine release is often coupled with bradykinin, is involved with allergic reactions, and is active in nasal, sinus, lung, skin and intestinal end organs.

Homocysteine: A sticky vascular inflammatory free radical that has similar properties to small particle LDL cholesterol. It can attach to membrane surfaces, plume inflammation, disrupt membrane function and induce chronic inflammation. Homocysteine levels increases with age and therefore intensify their proinflammatory effects on membrane surfaces. Elevated blood homocysteine levels are directly linked to increasing dementia and Parkinson Syndrome.

Homeostasis: In any given moment of time a cell is constantly adjusting to prevailing influences that are interacting with its function. Cellular homeostasis is optimized when chronic inflammation within interstitial spaces is suppressed. Thus the antithesis to capillary and end organ homeostasis is the constantly moving proinflammatory target of progressive chronic interstitial space inflammation and the disease venues it propagates.

Hydrostatic Pressure: Is the tension generated on endothelia based on the speed and force of blood flow through the lumen of a blood vessel. It is reflective of the rate and force of heart muscle contraction, the presence of basement membrane thickening or obstructive, the volume of blood in the vascular tree, and the net effects of inflammatory mediators on large vessel smooth muscle.

Hypertension: Is a disease venue brought about by basement membrane thickening as a result of accumulated vascular inflammatory free radicals. The increased *shear injury* to endothelia outer membranes from elevated blood pressures is in itself a vascular inflammatory free radical. So vascular free inflammatory radicals (such as smoke hydrocarbons, LDL cholesterol etc.) induce hypertension and the subsequent effect of increased shear stress on endothelia further perpetuate it. It is now defined as blood pressures of 130/85 or greater as taken by a sphygmomanometer cuff over proximal arm.

Hydrogen peroxide: Another toxic free radical exhaust product of mitochondrial energy combustion.

Hydroxynitriles: Are mitochondrial exhaust free radicals product from nitric oxide production. As capillary mitochondria get stuck in energy combustion from chronic inflammatory effects within the interstitial space, end organ mitochondria get stuck in nitric oxide combustion. The accumulation of hydroxynitriles within the end organ (which include cyanide) can be just as toxic as the accumulation of superoxide free radicals in capillaries and endothelia.

Hypoxic-Ischemic Event: Is a disease venue brought about by chronic inflammation within interstitial spaces and involves combinations of endothelial or capillary cell basement membrane disruption, accumulation of white blood cells, clotting factors and platelets, and the development of a thrombosis or occlusion. This cuts off blood flow and oxygen delivery to the end organ, which can lead to sudden compromise or even death to affected cells. Generally the larger the vessel involved, the more devastating to the end organ. In addition to thrombosis, other serious vascular occlusions can occur from emboli (where clot breaks off and travels upstream to occlude a smaller vessel) or plaque rupture (where the mature obstructive plaque explodes from within to release magnitudes of inflammatory debris upstream.

ICAMs, CAMS or capillary cell adhesion molecules: Are vast networks of specialized receptors on capillary cell outer membranes that include selectins, integrins and cadherin receptors among others. They are exposed and activated on the basis of different blends of protein kinase switches by cytokine signals which then cause adherence of choreographed white blood cells. These cells are rolled to the gap junction orifice where they enter the gap junction channel and are then further nuanced into the interstitial space staging area.

Immune Arsenal: Consist of cytokines, white blood cells, immunoglobulins, complement and platelets. They are also known as second line inflammatory mediators as they are part of our innate immunity. They expand the inflammatory response within interstitial spaces in order to eliminate inflammatory breach. With chronic inflammation in control of the interstitial space, their purpose shifts as they expand the inflammatory response to enable disease venues.

Immunoglobulins: A family of 5 different large proteins that are produced by different white blood cells. They represent a second arm of response to inflammatory breach (as opposed to the neutrophil-inducer-helper T lymphocyte arm). IgG and IGM are produced in bone marrow plasma cells and circulate widely within the blood stream whereas the other three immunoglobulins (IGA, IgD, IgE) are found in higher concentrations within sinuses, nose, lungs, skin and intestines.

Inducer- T Lymphocytes: Are white blood cells, along with neutrophils are choreographed early arrivers to the interstitial space staging area. As they assess and attack the inflammatory breach, they release important cytokines back to capillary cell outer membranes which further nuance additional staging. These signals will call out for more neutrophils, inducer lymphocytes or immunoglobulins, or will signal capillary cell outer membrane CAMs to attach next stage helper-lymphocytes or monocytes into the staging area.

Infectious agents: Are a disease venue defined as hostile foreign agents that take up residence within interstitial spaces and produce an inflammatory response, and often require additional outside treatment (ie., antibiotics) for the immune arsenal to regain control of the situation. The risk for infections increases when vascular inflammatory free radicals are abundant within the interstitial space or other disease venues such as diabetes, cancer or scarring are also occurring. Infectious agents include bacteria, viruses, fungus, parasites, amoebas and worms among others.

Insomnia: A condition that diminishes the capacity to fall or stay asleep. Insomnia can be due to anxiety, drugs (caffeine, stimulants), depression, psychosis, dementia, menopause, thyroid disorders, heart failure, COPD, prostate conditions, or overactive bladder, obesity, GERD (reflux of acid into the esophagus) or obstructive sleep apnea. It commonly is linked to sleep deprivation, which together can induce increases in vascular inflammatory free radicals through increases in released stress hormones and secondary behaviors associated with overeating and addictions.

Insulin Resistance or Pre Diabetes: Is defined as increases in fasting blood sugars between 100-125mg/dl and hemoglobin A1C levels from 5.8-6.4. It is considered a precursor to adult diabetes unless dietary changes, weight loss and exercise are implemented.

Interferons: A family of cytokines that have antiviral properties.

Integrins: A family of receptors on capillary cell outer membranes that are part of the CAM adhesion network.

Inter-endothelial Junction proteins or IEJ Proteins: Are proteins within the tight gap junction between capillary and endothelial cells that help pace and choreographed white blood cell trafficking into the interstitial space staging area.

Interleukin 1 or IL1: An early released proinflammatory cytokine (along with IL-6) that expands the inflammatory response within interstitial spaces.

Interleukin 6 or IL6: An early released proinflammatory cytokine released by white blood cells that expands the immune arsenal response to inflammatory breach.

Interleukin 10 or IL10: A potent anti-inflammatory cytokine that signals mop-op or completion of the inflammatory response. By inhibiting activity of T lymphocytes, monocytes and macrophages, IL-10 becomes and important signal to capillary outer membranes to downshift permeability to immune e arsenal trafficking and pendulum swing combustion to nitric oxide.

Interleukin T Helper Cells: A lymphocyte that secretes cytokines to mediate inflammation.

Interstitial Space: The space that separates the capillary cell basement membrane from those of the end organ. Interstitial space sanitation enables the capillary cell to optimally manage end organ signals calling for more oxygen or energy substrate. It is also the space where chronic inflammation can establish a foothold and initiate disease venues.

Junctional Adhesion Proteins or JAMS: Adhesion molecules within the tight gap junction that pace and select specific lymphocyte choreography into the interstitial space staging area.

Kallikreins: Circulating proteins, synthesized in the liver that are precursors to bradykinin.

Kinases: These are outer membrane protein enzymes that act as switches, can be induced by different cytokines, are responsive to reductions in membrane cAMP, and support exposures of different CAM receptors while biasing reductions in outer membrane voltage gradients. Protein kinase switches help to activate transport of inflammatory mediators via vesicles or transcellular channels.

Lactose: A disaccharide simple sugar (galactose plus glucose) that is not sweet, is found in dairy products, and can cause symptoms such as crampy abdominal pain, nausea, and bloating from an inability to breakdown the sugar. *Lactose intolerance* may increase with aging, and likely represents a spectrum of disease with varying symptoms that include predisposition to leaky gut.

Laminin: A family of glycoproteins that form part of the scaffolding of endothelial and capillary cell outer membranes.

LDL cholesterol also known as low density lipoprotein cholesterol, small particle LDL or oxidized LDL cholesterol: Is an inflammatory cholesterol produced in the liver. Once produced, it enters the blood plasma. It is lipid soluble meaning it is prone to traverse endothelial and capillary cell membrane surfaces to enter the interstitial space and attach to the basement membrane. Once attached, unless removed and degraded by HDL cholesterol, it will expand immune arsenal inflammation towards it. Along with other vascular inflammatory free radicals, it will cause eventual thickening of the basement membrane. Overtime this could lead to obstructive plaque on the membrane and a separation of the capillary's relationship to the end organ it serves. With obesity, diabetes, sarcopenia and inactivity, LDL cholesterol levels increase as HDL levels decrease.

Leaky Gut: A chronic inflammatory condition within the intestines producing malabsorption and caused by a deteriorating microbiome from highly refined white flour and sugar diets. Toxic nutrient gets advanced towards the portal circulation while good nutrient "leaks back" into the intestinal lumen and is non- absorbed.

Ligands: Usually a negatively charged molecule that binds to a positively charge cation or metal on a membrane surface to enable facilitated diffusion The binding is called a ligand and becomes a secondary messenger to the facilitated diffusion of electrolytes or other molecules across membrane surfaces.

Lipopolysaccharides: Also known as *LPS or endotoxins* are produced by gram negative bacteria that have infected an interstitial space and have spilled into the blood stream. When LPS is released, it becomes a potent inflammatory mediator that dramatically expands the inflammatory response and may induce fever, hypotension and multi-organ shutdown is a process known as sepsis.

Lipoprotein (a): A circulating sticky inflammatory LDL-like cholesterol that can snake its way through membrane surfaces and bind to the basement membrane or other membranes within the interstitial spaces of end organs. Elevated lipo(a) is linked can be inherited and is linked to premature heart attacks, aortic valve stenosis, strokes, dementia and other premature vascular events. It is treated with 2 grams daily of niacin or L-carnitine.

Lipoproteins: Proteins that have fatty acid constituents. They are found on membrane surfaces and bias mobilization of molecules through them that are lipid soluble. Lipoproteins can also act facilitate molecular transport via active transport or facilitated diffusion.

Luminal: Meaning an endothelial or capillary cell outer membrane directly exposed to circulating blood plasma.

Lymphokines: Are cytokines released from lymphocytes.

Lipoxins: A family of leukotrienes (cytokines) that cascade *resolvins* as a result of HEPE production and release by endothelial and capillary outer membranes. Lipoxins signal a turning point to inflammatory expansion within the interstitial space, implying an imminent pivot of reduced capillary cell outer membrane permeability, reduced trafficking of immune arsenal, and a swinging of mitochondrial combustion towards nitric oxide.

Lipoxygenase(s): Lipoxygenase enzymes **in** white blood cells convert arachidonic acid to proinflammatory cytokines (leukotrienes) that expand inflammation.

Lysosomes: Are budded from the Golgi apparatus. In the capillary cytoplasm they breakdown and and remove potentially toxic molecules.

Macrophages: Engulf and digest (phagocytize)processed inflammatory debris. They are part of the mesenchymal cell network within interstitial spaces.

MAPK also known as Mitogen Activated Protein Kinase: Is a protein kinase switch that is activated by growth factors to induce possible angiogenesis, mitosis and replication.

Mast Cells: A special type of white blood cell found within interstitial spaces of sinuses, nose, lung, and intestinal tract. Mast cells contain granules composed of histamine and heparin. When released, this can substantially increase an inflammatory (allergic) response.

Melanocytes: A special type of mesenchymal cell within the skin.

Monocyte Chemotactic Factors (MCFs): A family of enzymes released by monocytes, and includes MCP-1. When released, MCFs signal endothelial and capillary cells to send from blood plasma additional T lymphocytes and mononuclear cells to the interstitial space staging area.

MCP-1 also known as Monocyte Chemotactic Protein-1 or Cytokine A2: This molecule is elevated within interstitial spaces in chronic inflammatory disease venues including adult diabetes, obesity, metabolic syndrome and hypoxia-ischemia. When released it tells capillary cells to increase T-lymphocytes and monocytes into the interstitial space staging area. Like most cytokines, when properly choreographed by capillary cells, MCP-1 becomes critical piece to the elimination of vascular inflammatory free radicals or other types of inflammatory breach. In the setting of chronic inflammation, MCP-1 can become a malignant foe as its chronic release coupled with capillary cell outer membrane pseudocapillarization enables expansion of wayward T lymphocytes and monocytes into the staging area. It becomes just a matter of time before a white blood cell led coupe occurs utilizing an increasing hostile feedback loop signaling cascade with little or no resistance from the disabled capillary cells.

Medical Industrial Complex: Is an expensive conglomerate or expensive tests, procedures and treatments utilized in an ever increasing complex way to manage the exponential explosion of different disease venues. Many agree that further escalation of disease treatment without attempting to reverse vascular inflammatory risks will bankrupt western cultures sooner rather than later.

Medicinals: Are disease treatments that have approved FDA indications. Medicinals are considered allopathic prescriptions for the treatment of specific conditions. They may or may not influence inflammation. For this reason many medicinals, while treating diseases, could make underlying interstitial space inflammation worse. Examples include certain medications to treat GERD (esophageal reflex), all stimulant ADHD drugs, and many antidepressant and antipsychotic drugs.

Mesenchymal Cells: A basket of cells that reside within the interstitial spaces of end organs that help frame and inflammatory response to an interstitial space inflammatory breach. Examples of different mesenchymal cells include pericytes and astrocytes of the blood brain barrier and Kupffer and stellate cells in the liver sinusoid.

Microbiome: Composes the bacterial population within the intestinal lumen. The microbiome will change based on diet. A healthy microbiome is integral to optimal intestinal nutrient absorption and becomes optimal in diets of large quantities of organic whole food plant fiber.

Microfilaments: Are actin- myosin attachments to the capillary cell continuous outer membrane and cytoplasm infrastructure. These microfilaments affect outer membrane configuration and the widening or narrowing of the gap junction orifice and channel, thus enabling control of pace to immune arsenal entry into the interstitial space.

Microtubules: Connect the continuous outer membrane of the capillary cell to the centriole-centrosome complex. When stimulated by growth factors, the microtubule connection facilitates the capillary cell's ability to divide into two cells to potentially form new blood vessels.

Microvilli: Are caverns on capillary cell continuous outer membrane which enables potential exposure to more receptors. Because they are cavernous their receptors can be protected from hostile outside forces that include shear stress.

Mitochondria: Capillary cell mitochondria supply up to 15% of endothelial cell energy but it is there pivot and swing of combustion from energy to nitric oxide based on outer membrane permeability adjustments that makes them critical to interstitial space sanitation and end organ function. With chronic inflammation within interstitial spaces, endothelial and capillary cell mitochondrial volumes get depleted, which is directly linked to outer membrane pseudocapillarization and an increasingly incompetent nuclear DNA.

Monokines: Are cytokines released by monocytes that signal late stages of inflammatory breach elimination.

Mucopolysaccharides: Unbranched complex carbohydrates or polysaccharides of repeating disaccharides or simple sugars. Mucopolysaccharides are also known as glycosaminoglycans or GAGS. Mucopolysaccharides are concentrated in mucous membranes and in joint spaces. When part of a disease venue, they may contribute to sinus infections, bronchitis, pneumonias and joint pain (arthritis).

Myeloperoxidases: A heme containing enzyme, found in monocytes and neutrophil granules that acts as an antioxidant to break down hydrogen peroxide free radical to carbon dioxide and water.

Myosin Light Chain Kinase and Myosin Light Chain Phosphatase also known as MLCK, and MLCP Are endothelial and capillary cell outer membrane switches that can be activated by inflammatory mediators, such as thrombin, histamine and bradykinin to induce among other things actin-myosin filament sliding.

NAD (Nicotinamide Adenine Dinucleotide): Like FAD (Flavin adenine dinucleotide), NAD is found in high concentrations within mitochondria, and both FAD and NAD serve as hydrogen ion transporters. They pick up hydrogen ions from pyruvate and beta oxidation as well as from the Krebs cycle and deposit them into cytochromes I-III to facilitate electron transfer. The process or supplying hydrogen to the cytochromes supports the inner membrane electromechanical voltage gradient and provides an abundant source of hydrogen for the final stage of converting ADP to ATP.

Nitric Oxide: A powerful gas that is produced primarily by mitochondrial combustion. It becomes the gas of capillary and endothelial cell cellular rejuvenation and is blatantly reduced in chronic interstitial space inflammation. Capillary cell nitric oxide production also increases blood flow, oxygen, and nutrient to the end organ thereby optimizing end organ function. It serves as a powerful feedback loop to mesenchymal cells to stimulate their rejuvenation as well as a stimulus to end organ mitochondria to combust more energy. In this sense nitric oxide production and the feedback loops it generates drives quality assurance to the capillary cell and its partners. The production of nitric oxide gas is dependent on a downshift in permeability to immune arsenal trafficking, which becomes dependent on the volume of vascular inflammatory free radical fuel that is impinging the interstitial space.

Nucleus: The "brain" of the capillary cell that contains the genetic code (on chromosomes) for protein synthesis to replicate and repair most of the cell's outer membranes and infrastructure. Integral to the coding process is the nucleolus, which resides inside the nucleus, makes up 35% of nuclear volume and is responsible for nuclear transcription of the DNA to messenger RNA. The messenger RNA is then mobilized to ribosomes and the rough endoplasmic reticulum to initiate protein synthesis, usually under the auspice of mitochondrial combustion of nitric oxide. With aging or chronic interstitial space inflammation the telomere cap that protects nuclear chromosomal DNA shrinks enabling more DNA to be exposed to free radical cross linkage. Damaged DNA either silences or disrupts the production of normal proteins.

Omega Three Fatty Acids: Are primarily EPA (eicosapentaenoic acid) and DHA (docosahexaenoic acid) chain react multiple anti-inflammatory effects in endothelia. When utilized as a substrate by different enzymes, instead of arachidonic acid, they cascade feedback loops that signal reductions in interstitial space inflammation.

Oncotic Pressure: A pressure gradient on a membrane generated by the difference in albumin concentrations on one side of the membrane compared to the other. The gradient favors pulling water and electrolytes across the membrane surface where there is more albumin thereby *dehydrating* the side of the membrane where there is less albumin..

Opsonization: A process of breaking down a foreign invader or free radical initiated by an immunoglobulin plus complement (antigen –antibody complex) or complement alone. Effective opsonization leads to monocyte or macrophage phagocytosis (engulfment)

Outer Membranes: All cells in the human body have outer membranes which serve to protect the cells infrastructure and support specific cell function. The vascular endothelium and specifically the capillary cell have a very unique set of outer membranes that are composed of a very dense receptor network. The receptor network enables precise choreography of immune arsenal intent within the interstitial space. The capillary outer membrane network consists of a luminal glycocalyx, continuous outer membrane and abluminal basement membrane. Whereas the glycoalcyx supports choreography to intestinal space breach, the basement membrane optimizes specific function of the end organ it serves.

PAI-1 or plasminogen Activator Inhibitor: Blocks tissue plasminogen activator (also known as tPA), which biases thrombosis and hypoxic ischemic events.

PARS 1 or protease activated receptor-1: A family of 4 different receptors that mediate the effects of thrombin attachment. The *PARS-1-thrombin* capillary cell membrane attachment produces increases permeability trafficking of immune arsenal into interstitial spaces in addition to increasing proclotting biases. In contrast to bradykinin, Pars-1-thrombin complex will cause arteriole smooth muscle contraction thereby reducing blood flow to upstream capillary beds and potentially placing end organs at risk for hypoxic- ischemic events.

Particulates: Small particles that when persistently inhaled (such as from tobacco smoke), can cause chronic inflammation within the interstitial spaces of the lung. Inhaling particulates is often associated with inhaling other toxic resides thereby magnifying toxic effects. Particulates can be noxious gases, dust, air pollution, toxic fumes, or residues from animal fur, birds, farm animals, asbestos, insecticides or pesticides.

Passive Transport: The process where molecules, such as gases, are moved through membranes without energy. Gas or electrolyte movement is based on *gradients or gas tensions* on one side of the membrane compared to the other. When a gas is of higher concentration on one side of the membrane it will passively move across the membrane to equilibrate.

Paxillin: A membrane infrastructure protein that is linked to FAK (focal adhesion kinase-switch). It can assist in nuancing different CAM exposures.

Pericytes: A type of mesenchymal cell within the interstitial space of different end organs. In the brain, they form a partnership with astrocytes and capillaries to form the blood brain barrier.

Platelet Derived Growth Factor or PDGF: Along with VEGF, can stimulate the growth of new blood vessels, usually in response to end organ hypoxia or acute and chronic interstitial space inflammation.

Platelet Endothelial cell Adhesion Molecule (also known as PECAM-1): A family of proteins within the tight gap junction that attaches platelets to limit the pace of choreographed white blood cells trafficking through the gap unction. This block becomes important when cytokine signals from mesenchymal and monocytes within the interstitial space call for mop –up operations and closure of the inflammatory response.

Perlecan: A glycoprotein within the capillary cell basement membrane infrastructure that is additive to barrier function, as might be seen in capillary cells of the blood brain barrier.

Permeability: Refers to capillary and endothelial cell outer membrane's capacity to adjust trafficking of immune arsenal into and out of the interstitial space. Effective permeability adjustment requires a full complement of outer membrane receptors and a capable volume of mitochondria. Those requisites become dependent on limiting vascular inflammatory free radical breach into the interstitial space. This enables the capillary cell outer membranes to pivot and then signal a swinging of mitochondrial combustion from energy to nitric oxide.

Peroxisomes: Manufactured by ribosomes, they are situated close to capillary cell outer membranes and encapsulate large chain fatty acids that have penetrated the cytoplasm and proceed to break them down to smaller fatty acid chains, which can then enter the mitochondria and participate in beta oxidation. Peroxisomes can also help decompose toxic fatty acids.

Phospholipases (or commonly known as the Phospholipase C Family of Enzymes): A group of 13 different enzymes found in most cells. Within endothelial and capillary cell outer membranes they facilitate oxidation (breakdown) of phospholipids and complex fatty acids to simpler forms.

Plasma Membrane: Describes the endothelial and capillary cell continuous outer membrane that is on the luminal side of the cell.

Pleotropic Effect: Is used to describe cascading effects that were not otherwise anticipated from a treatment or intervention. As an example aspirin, by blocking production of thromboxane in platelets reduces their adhesion to decrease risks for thrombosis. What was not anticipated is how this effect cascades to reduce cancers throughout the intestinal tract. A similar case can be made for statins and their known effect in reducing LDL cholesterol and subsequent development of obstructive plaque and risk for occlusive thrombosis. What is not expected is its beneficial effects in reducing many different cancers, infections, atrial fibrillation etc.

Pluming of Inflammation: A process where inflammatory momentum within the interstitial space expands.

PPARs also known as Peroxisome Proliferator Activator Receptors: Are receptors found in nuclear membranes that regulate the expression of genes. PPAR receptors can be considered anti-inflammatory receptors as they reduce insulin resistance thereby improving blood sugar management. The PPAR-DHA complex can serve as an antioxidant.

Prostacyclin also known as PGI-2: Is produced from prostaglandins in capillary and endothelial cells, and produces similar relaxing effects on smooth muscle as nitric oxide. It facilitates increased blood flow to the capillary bed while also blocking platelet aggregation within the interstitial space or on the luminal membrane surface. Both of these properties favorably impact end organs (brain, heart cornea) that are heavily dependent on oxygen delivery for their function. The antithesis to endothelial prostacyclin production is *endothelin* which has the opposite effect on smooth muscle and is biased to production from chronic inflammation. In capillary cells, pendulum swinging mitochondrial combustion to nitric oxide, favors prostacyclin production, which is associated with decreased activation of proinflammatory mediators - VEGF, TGF, and interleukins 1 and 6.

Prostaglandins: A diverse family of fatty acids which contain a 5 carbon ring and are found in all cells Prostaglandin end products in endothelia, depending on prevailing cytokine signals, can be prostacyclin (which is anti-inflammatory) and thromboxane (proinflammatory).

Protease Enzymes: Enzymes that break down (catabolize) proteins into smaller constituent molecules.

Protectins: Produced by neutrophils (along with resolvins as part of a feedback loop signal with endothelia and capillary cells) to signal termination or blunting of an inflammatory response.

Protein Kinase A, also known as PKA: Are families of membrane switches that are linked to cAMP activity and bias reductions in outer membrane permeability. PKA activation reduces outer membrane permeability whereas the *protein kinase C* (PKC) family of membrane switches biases increases in membrane permeability. The *cAMP-protein kinase A* driven outer membrane permeability pivot becomes a critical to long term capillary cell viability as it enables the swinging of mitochondrial combustion from energy to nitric oxide.

Proteoglycans : A glycoprotein found in cellular membrane including endothelial and capillary cell outer membrane infrastructure

Pseudocapillarization: Is a destructive outcome to capillary cell outer membranes due to the persistent effects of chronic interstitial space inflammation. Along with reduced mitochondrial volumes and increased nuclear DNA damage, pseudocapillarization of capillary cell outer membranes includes lost receptor volumes, diminished voltage gradients and reduces pore diversity, all of which favor a more random and mistake prone immune arsenal entry into the interstitial space.

RAGE (also known as Receptor for Advanced Glycation End Products) : Becomes activated on endothelial and capillary cell outer membranes by the presence of the free radical AGE (advanced glycation end product). The AGE to RAGE activation increases with diabetes and sugar ingestion as it cascades inflammatory expansion within interstitial spaces by increasing capillary cell permeability trafficking of inflammatory mediators.

RANTES (also known as CCL-5 or Regulated on Activation Normal T Cell Expressed and Secreted): A cytokine that attracts memory T cells and monocytes from blood or lymph as part of an expressed capillary cell choreography in the latter stages of interstitial space breach elimination. .

Replication: A process that begins in the nucleus where DNA is copied in preparation for protein synthesis or mitosis. *Transcription* is when the DNA is copied to messenger RNA. Messenger RNA then travels to ribosomes and rough endoplasmic reticulum the copied code is translated into protein synthesis.

Resolvins: Produced by neutrophils to signal mop-up of an inflammatory response.

Rho Proteins: Are small protein switches on membrane surfaces that are linked to the GTPase enzymes that release energy as GTP gets converted to GDP. The conversion becomes a second cascading energy energy source to ATP. Rho proteins include the subfamilies of *RhoA, RAC, ROCK and CDC 42.* These activated receptors nuance increases in endothelial and capillary cell outer membrane permeability by facilitating exposures of CAM receptors for choreographed immune arsenal attachment.

Rough Endoplasmic Reticulum: Contain ribosomes which together form manufacturing units for translating mRNA into protein synthesis. Rough ER should not be confused with **smooth endoplasmic reticulum**, which is linked to mitochondrial storage and release of calcium ions and the production and storage of heme.

Sarcopenia: Age related loss of skeletal muscle mass and tone increasing risk for falls and adult diabetes.

Scar tissue: Can be beneficial as part of healing a wound. In chronic inflammatory conditions within the interstitial space of end organs, scar tissue becomes a disease venue which separates the capillary cell from the end organ. It is usually secreted by mesenchymal cells, which in the setting of chronic inflammation, are responding to rogue feedback loop signals generated by rebel white blood cells.

Second- Line Vascular Inflammatory Mediators: Are known as our innate immune arsenal respond to inflammatory breach. They are in contrast to *first- line inflammatory mediators*, which are vascular inflammatory free radicals.

Seeding Inflammation: A term used to describe how a vascular inflammatory free radical penetrates through endothelial cells from the blood plasma, emerges into the interstitial space, attaches to a membrane surface and then attracts immune arsenal towards it to expand inflammation.

Selectin Receptors: Are families of adhesion receptors (CAMs) on capillary cell outer membranes that facilitate the rolling of white blood cells towards the gap junction orifice.

Selective Permeability of Inflammatory Mediators: Is the equivalent of a sequenced or choreographed immune arsenal trafficking into interstitial spaces in the management of sanitation and elimination of inflammatory breach.

Serum Amyloid A: A family of proinflammatory proteins produced in the liver and circulate in the blood stream and are linked to large arterial vessel obstructive plaque, chronic infections or autoimmune complex diseases.

Shear Stress: When blood pressures increase from accumulations of vascular inflammatory free radicals on endothelial basement membranes, the vessel stiffens and becomes less responsive to smooth muscle thereby increasing shear stress and endothelial cell injury.

Sirtuins: A family of a least 7 proteins found in most cells that when activated, bias anti-inflammatory momentum while reducing the effects of prediabetes or diabetes. Sirtuint 1 is found in the nucleus whereas sirtuins 3-5 are found in mitochondria. Supplements that activate sirtuins reduce insulin resistance, prevent certain infections and lengthen life span. When capillary cell mitochondria are combusting energy, sirtuins 3-5 are deactivated. On the other hand, when nitric oxide is being produced, sirtuin activity is increased.

Sleep Deprivation: A serious condition where there is failure to obtain at least 7 hours of sleep. It causes are multifactorial.

Smooth Muscle Cells: Are found throughout the body and in different end organs. They compose the end organ to large vessel arteries down to the arteriole. These cells are signaled to contract or relax to constrict or expand the vessel lumen to decrease or increase blood flow through the vessel lumen. Chronic inflammation within the endothelial cell's interstitial space, thickens the basement membrane, reduces communication signals to the smooth muscle, and lessens the smooth muscle's capacity to impact signaling influences, thereby biasing reductions in blood flow.

Somatic Cells: Are epithelial derived cells that differentiate into an end organ.

Sphingosines: Are produced in lysosomes when sphingolipid is degraded to sphingosine. Sphingosine-1 phosphate is produced from sphingosine.

Sphingosine-1 Phosphate (also known as S1P): Can be considered a cytokine, that when released by white blood cells, binds to up to capillary and endothelial cell outer membrane G (EDG) receptors to decrease permeability. In this sense S1P provides mop-up anti-inflammatory momentum that could be coordinated with protectins and resolvins. S1P activated EDG receptors block further penetration of migrating T cells into the interstitial space. This action would serve notice to pendulum swing capillary cell mitochondrial combustion to nitric oxide thereby shuttling mitochondrial acetyl coenzyme A away from Krebs cycle and towards ribosomes to facilitate repair, replacement and replication of proteins. When the interstitial space is controlled by chronic inflammation, released S-1P blocks T lymphocyte migration into the interstitial space thereby causing immune suppression and enabling the dissemination of cancers cells or infectious agents.

SRC Families (also known as Steroid Receptor Coactivator): Serves as an endothelial and capillary cell outer membrane switch, as its activation uncouples phosphorus from ATP to release energy. In this manner, it acts similarly to how Rho releases energy at the membrane by uncoupling phosphorus from GTP. Activation of either the SRC or Rho families implies increased energy utilization at endothelial and capillary outer membrane surfaces meaning that active transport of inflammatory mediators into the interstitial space is occurring. In chronic inflammation, SRC and Rho switches are chronically activated.

Stacking Inflammation: Is caused when there is clustering of vascular inflammatory free radicals into interstitial spaces of end organs, thereby accelerating inflammatory expansion and perpetrating chronic inflammatory risk.

Stem Cells: Immature progenitor cells that can replicate mature cells or parts of mature cells. Stem cells are being used to treat chronic inflammatory conditions.

Superoxide: A toxic free radical exhaust (or *ROS-reactive oxygen species*) product of mitochondrial combustion to make energy. Excessive superoxide exhaust spearheads DNA damage in endothelial and capillary cells thereby chain reacting a sequence of events leading to reduced mitochondrial volumes and pseudocapillarization of outer membranes.

Supplements: Are vitamins, minerals, enzymes, fatty acids or plant based complex carbohydrates that can be purchased over the counter and have anti-inflammatory properties. They generally have no FDA approved indications for disease treatment. They are poorly regulated and often over exaggerate their effectiveness making the medical establishment resistant to their use. Since they are unregulated, dosing them is often a best guess and their quality from one manufacturer to the next is dubious. Nevertheless, in the elderly and chronically infirmed, supplements can improve deficiency states and are additive to lifestyle adjustments.

Symport: Is an energy driven sodium pump that keeps continuous outer membrane sodium concentrations higher in their cytoplasm, thereby facilitating an increase membrane voltage gradient. This becomes favorable to reducing outer membrane permeability to immune arsenal trafficking and is associated with increased levels of membrane cAMP. The symport mechanics of sodium pumping into the cytoplasm often carries vagabond attachments with the transported sodium. In this manner, the cytoplasm gets two for the price of one.

Talin: A endothelial–capillary cell infrastructure membrane protein that can assist in choreography to expose specific CAMs for white blood cell attachment.

Telomere Cap: Is manufactured by telomerase and is responsible for protecting nuclear chromosomal DNA from free radical cross linkage. The telomere cap shrinks quickly when there is chronic interstitial space inflammation, making chromosomal DNA at risk for free radical damage. The cross linkage silences protein synthesis and predisposes to reduced capillary cell mitochondrial volumes and pseudocapillarization of outer membranes.

Tensin: A capillary continuous outer membrane infrastructure protein that can reconfigure to expose choreographed CAM receptors for white blood cell attachment.

Tight Gap Junction: Refers to a specific location within the gap junction where white blood cell trafficking is nuanced. A tight gap junction could also refer to a compacted and narrow gap junction channel, seen in capillaries of the blood brain or blood optic nerve barrier.

Toxins: A term used to connote any molecule that potentially disrupts cellular or interstitial space homeostasis. Toxins become problematic with lifestyle choices that involve addictions to drugs, alcohol or nicotine or from recurrent adverse environmental exposures.

Thrombin: Also known as clotting factor II or IIA. When activated, thrombin converts fibrinogen to fibrin to form a clot. Like all clotting factors it is produced in the liver and is part of the clotting cascade. This is beneficial in situations where there is trauma or bleeding, but with chronic inflammation, pro clotting biases increase risk clotting mistakes that can create dire end organ outcomes.

Thromboxanes: Are manufactured from prostaglandins and cascade proinflammatory momentum. With chronic inflammation, endothelial cells produce more thromboxane from prostaglandins then prostacyclin. Thromboxane A2 is a potent vasoconstrictor as well as an inducer of platelet aggregation which promotes clotting and thrombosis. In the setting of chronic inflammation, it leads to strokes and heart attacks that culminate in heart failure and dementia. Daily doses of aspirin (81 milligrams) blocks thromboxane from causing thrombosis which limits these serious adverse outcomes.

Transcytosis: A transport process where a molecule is trafficked through the cells cytoplasm via a vesicle or transport channel. Transport can go both ways, from interstitial space to blood plasma or visa-versa.

Triglycerides: A circulating proinflammatory free radical manufactured by fat cells. When triglyceride levels are elevated the blood plasma gets milky and the triglyceride can incorporate into endothelial outer membranes to disrupt infrastructure and receptor function. They may also get into the cell and bias increases in gluconeogenesis thereby increasing insulin resistance.

Trans-Fats: Highly inflammatory fat molecule composed of polyunsaturated carbon rings (vegetable oils) that reconfigure from cis to trans from heat or light exposure. Reconfiguration enables trans-fats to enter into membranes and disable their infrastructure.

Transforming Growth Factor (TGF-beta): A family of cytokine growth factor that are produced by a variety of cells in proinflammatory conditions within interstitial spaces. When part of a choreographed inflammatory response, TGF- beta can help expand the inflammatory response to eliminate inflammatory breach. If induced by rogue influences, its production escalates risk for disease venues.

Tumor Necrosis Factor (also known as TNF-alpha, cachexin or cachectin): Produced by a variety of cells as a proinflammatory cytokine that expands inflammation. When sequenced properly it participates in inflammatory breach elimination. When expressed chronically, it promotes disease venues.

Tyrosine Kinases: A family of membrane switches which increase capillary outer membrane permeability to immune arsenal trafficking. Some protein kinases can activate VEGF, which modulates the expression of new blood vessel growth. Depending on what controls the interstitial space, activated VEGF can work for or against interstitial space sanitation and the best interests of the end organ.

Vascular Inflammatory Mediator- Risks: Are first-line inflammatory mediators that are free radicals, that often lifestyle generated. They mobilize into interstial sapces, often in stealth and attach to outer membranes including the basement membrane to expand inflammation by attracting immune arsenal l towards them. As such they serve as fuel for chronic inflammation. They include AGEs from sugar, LDL cholesterol, non HDL cholesterol, triglycerides, lipo (a), homocysteine, cigarette toxins, toxic gases including carbon monoxide), pesticides, insecticides, inhaled particulates, drugs and alcohol. They can be further aggravated by stress hormones, overeating, inactivity and sleep deprivation.

Vacuoles: Storage "bubbles" in the cell. When vacuoles are lysosomes, they facilitate breakdown of intracellular toxins. .

VEGF or Vascular endothelial growth factor: Is produced from a variety of different cells, including the capillary and endothelial cells. It is one of several growth factors that can induce cellular mitosis (cell division), or in the case of capillary cells, angiogenesis.

Vesicle and Vacuole Organelle (also known as VVO(s)): Intracellular vacuoles that in endothelia provide mechanics to transport of large bulky molecules back into the blood plasma.

Vesicles: Are active transport vehicles, often formed from outer membrane caveolae, that move larger molecules, such as albumin, from the blood plasma through the capillary cell's cytoplasm to be dispersed into the interstitial space.

Veniculin: A endothelial-capillary infrastructure outer membrane protein that when reconfigured, participates in the choreography of different CAM exposures for white blood cell attachment.

Water Soluble: A method of describing molecular solubility. A molecule that is more eater soluble will meet greater resistance towards penetrating the membrane than if it had more lipid (fat) solubility.

White Blood Cells: Are produced in the bone marrow and can circulate in the blood plasma or be stored in the bone marrow, lymph tissue and spleen. They respond to cytokine signaling where they mobilize to capillary cell outer membranes to be attached by CAM receptors and trafficked through the gap junction channel or occasionally transported by vesicles or transport channels. Choreography by capillary cell outer membranes enables white blood cell s to be paced and specifically staged into the interstitial space to eliminate inflammatory breach. White blood cells can subdivided into granulocyte cells, which are more immediate responders to inflammation, and lymphocytes, which include helper and inducer T cells, B cells and monocytes. Granulocytes include neutrophils, basophils and eosinophils. B cell lymphocytes include a family of 8 different cells involved in the expression of humoral antibodies. Many of these white blood cells responses in addition to endothelial and capillary cell choreography require additional signaling help from interstitial space macrophages or T lymphocytes.

Xanthine-Xanthine Oxidase Complex: A set of endothelial and capillary cell outer membrane receptors that can decrease cAMP levels, to facilitate cascades of proinflammatory momentum including activation of protein kinase activation and increases in CAM exposures.

Zyxin: A zinc containing endothelial and capillary cell infrastructure outer membrane protein that can reconfigure to express different CAM exposures.

APPENDIX

Graph 1: The Stacking of Vascular Inflammatory Free radicals, Poor Lifestyle Choices and Subsequent Disease Venues on Mortality (Courtesy of *Hazing Aging*, I Universe, 2015)

This graph demonstrates the relationship of circulating vascular inflammatory free radicals (ie. LDL cholesterol, non HDL cholesterol etc.), poor lifestyle choices (smoking cigarettes) and unmitigated disease venues (adult diabetes, hypertension) has on accelerating mortality. The implication in the graph, is that all of these risks impinge inflammatory risk on interstitial spaces, block the capillary cell pivot and swing dance, to nurture a coup of feedback loop control away from capillary cell choreography and towards wayward interstitial space white blood cells. Mortality increases from different disease venues that include disseminated cancer or infection, thrombosis, progressive end organ scarring or autoimmune complex disease.

Graph 2: The Effect of Aging on Sarcopenia, Circulating Advanced Glycation End Products (AGES) and Insulin Resistance

This graph demonstrates the relationship of Aging and how it biases loss of muscle mass and tone, increases the risk for sustained elevations in circulating advanced glycation end products and insulin resistance. The implication is that the effect of aging must be mitigated with a amore disciplined regimen involving reductions in simple sugar ingestion and regular aerobic and anaerobic exercise to restore muscle mass. It must also include intentional stress reduction and improved sleep hygiene. Eating one donut, smoking one cigarette or drinking one alcoholic beverage at age 65 may be the equivalent of three of the same at age 25 as to its effects on circulating vascular inflammatory free radicals..

Graph 3: The Causes and Effects of the Three Stages of Chronic Interstitial Space Inflammation and the Capillary Cell Fail

This graph highlights the three stages of chronic inflammation beginning with the impingement of interstitial spaces with vascular inflammatory free radicals at the far left of the graph. Their persistence coupled with the mounting inability to clear them from basement membranes and interstitial spaces, keeps capillary cell mitochondria stuck in energy combustion mode. This causes build-ups in superoxide ROS within the capillary cell, which eventually cross links DNA, silences certain protein synthesis and limits the capillary cell's capacity to replace, or repair its infrastructure, outer membranes or mitochondria. Mistakes are made in capillary cell choreography which include enabling wayward white blood cell entrance into the interstitial space. As these cells increase their presence within the interstitial space, they initiate signaling of cytokines which scramble capillary cell intent thereby enhancing rather than eliminating inflammatory breach. As these signals become the preferred feedback loop system within the interstitial space the capillary cell outer membranes are hijacked and the mesenchymal cells turned to favor the rogue feedback loop system. This defines the second stage of chronic inflammation defined as the *inflammatory matrix*. With the chronic inflammatory infrastructure now in place, disease venues can be initiated within the interstitial space with cancer and infectious agents taking on a life of their own in extension with the chronic inflammatory agenda. With the advent of disease venues, the maturing of chronic inflammation into the third stage has occurred and is known as *the anti-organ*. Current disease treatment models that dominate international medicine involve chronic inflammation at this late third stage.

BIBLIOGRAPHY

Abraham, D. and O. Distler," How does endothelial cell injury start? The role of endothelin in systemic sclerosis," *Arthritis Res Ther*, 2007,9(2):S2

Alghadir, A. H., S. A. Gabr and E. S. Al-Eisa," Effects of moderate aerobic exercise on cognitive abilities and redox state biomarkers in older adults," *Oxidative Medicine and Cellular Longevity*, 2016,(2016) 2545168,8pages.

Al-Soudi, A., M. H. Kaaij and S. W. Tas," Endothelial cells: from innocent bystanders to active participants in immune responses," *Autoimmunity Reviews*, 2017,16(9):951-962.

Bernatova, I.,"Endothelial dysfunction in experimental models of arterial hypertension: cause or consequence?" *Biomed Res Int*, 2014,10.1155/598271.

Buckingham, Robert. Hazing Aging: *How Capillary Endothelia Control Inflammation and Aging.* Bloomington, IN: I Universe, 2015.

Buckingham, Robert. Rejuvenation!: *How the Capillary Cell Dance Blocks Aging while Decreasing Pain and Fatigue.* Bloomington, IN: I Universe, 2107.

Cai, H. and D. G. Harrison," Endothelial dysfunction in cardiovascular diseases: the role of oxidant stress," *Circulation Research*, 2000(87):840-844.

Cheung, K., C.P. Ward, E. J. Fu. H and Marelli-Berg, and M. Federica," Endothelial cells:immunobiological aspects," *eLS*. John Wiley and Sons Ltd, http://www.els.net. Doi:10.1002/9780470015902.a00005 13.pub3. Top of Form

Danese, S., E. Dejana and C. Fiocchi," Immune regulation by microvascular endothelial cells: directing innate and adaptive immunity, coagulation and inflammation," *J Immunol*, 2007,178(10):6017-6022.

Davidson, S. M. and M. R. Duchen," Endothelial mitochondria contributing to vascular function and disease," *Circulation Research*, 2007,100,1128-1141.

Davignon, J. and R. Ganz," Role of endothelial dysfunction in Atheroslcerosis," *Circulation*, 2004,109:III27-32.

Egemnazarov, B., S. Cmkovic, B. M. Nagy, H Olschewski and G. Kwapiszewska," Right ventricular fibrosis and dysfunction:actual concepts and common misconception," *J Matbio*, 2018.01.010.

Favero, G., C. Paganelli, B. Buffoli, L. F. Rodella and R. Rezzani," Endothelium and its alterations in cardiovascular diseases: life style intervention,"*BioMed Research international*, 2014(2014),801896,28 pages.

Franses, J. W., N. C. Drosu, W. J. Gibson, V. C. Chitalia and E. R. Edelman," Dysfunctional endothelial cells directly stimulate cancer inflammation and metastasis," *Int. J. Cancer,*2013,133(6):1334-1344.

Gaengel, K., G. Genove, A. Armulik, and C. Betsholz," Endothelial-mural cell signaling in vascular development and angiogenesis," *Arteriosclerosis, Thrombosis, and Vascular Biology*, 2009,29:630-638.

Gao, Y., M. Bielohuby, T. Fleming, G.F. Grabner, E. Foppen, W. Bernhard, M. Guzman-Ruiz, C. Layritz, B. Legutko, E. Zinser, C. Garcia-Caceres, R. M. Buijs, S. C. Woods, A. Kalsbeek, R. J. Seeley, P. P. Nawroth, M. Bidlingmaier, M.H. Tschop, and C-X. Yi," Dietary sugars, not lipids, drive hypothalamic inflammation,"*Molmet*, 2017,6(8):897-908.

Goncharov, N. V., A. D. Nadeev, R. O. Jenkins and P. V. Avdonin," Markers and biomarkers of endothelium: when something is rotten in the state," *Oxidative Medicine and Cellular Longevity*, 2017(2017),9759735,27pages.

Goncharov, N. V., A.I. Ukolov, T. I. Orlova, E.D. Migolovskaia and N. G. Voitenko," Metabolomics: on the way to an integration of biochemistry, analytical chemistry and informatics," *Biology Bulletin Reviews*, 2015,5(4):296-307.

Granger, D.N. and E. Senchenkova, "Inflammation and the microcirculation," *Chapter 10, Endothelial Barrier Dysfunction*, :Morgan and Claypool Life Sciences, San Rafael (CA), 2010, http://www.ncbi.nlm.nih.gov/books.

Hallmark R., J. T. Patrie, Z. Liu, G. A. Gaesser, E. J. Barrett and A. Weltman, The effect of exercise intensity on endothelial function in physically inactive lean and obese adults. *PLoS ONE,*2014, 9(1):e85450.

Henderson, W. R.," The role of leukotrienes in inflammation," *Ann Int Med,* 1994,121(9):684-697.

Janus, A., E. Szahidewicz-Krupska, G. Majur, and A Doroszko,"Insulin resistance and endothelial dysfunction constitute a common therapeutic target in cardiometabolic disorders," *Mediators Inflamm,* 2016,doi:10.1155/2016/3634948.

Joshi, M., S. R. Kotha, S. Malireddi, V. Selvaraju, A. Satoskar, A. R. Satoskar, A. Palesty, D. W. McFadden, N. L. Parinandi and N. Maulik," Conundrum of pathogenesis of diabetic cardiomyopathy: role of vascular endothelial dysfunction, reactive oxygen species and mitochondria," *Molecular and Cellular Biochemistry*, 2014,386(1-2):233-249.

Khazaeia, F., I. Moien-afsharib and B Laher," Review vascular endothelial function in health and disease," *Pathophysiology*, 2008,15,49–67.

Kheirandish-Gozal, L., M.F. Philby, Z. Qiao, A. Khalyfa and D.Gozal," Endothelial dysfunction in children with obstructive sleep apnea is associated with elevated lipoprotein-associated phospholipase A2 plasma activity levels," *Journal of the American Heart Association*, 2017,6:e004923.

Kolka, C.M., and R.N. Bergman," The barrier within: endothelial transport of hormones," *Physiology*, 2012,27:237-247.

Kumar, A., C.W. Kim, R.D. Simmons and H. Jo," Rolfe of flow sensitive microRNAs in endothelial dysfunction and atherosclerosis-"mechanosensitive athero-mirs," *Arteriolscler Thromb Vasc Biol*, 2014,34(10):2206-2216.

Kumar, P., Y. Ning and P. J. Polverini," Endothelial cell expressing Bcl-2 promotes tumor metastasis by enhancing tumor angiogenesis, blood vessel leakiness and tumor invasion," *Lab Invest,*2008,88(7):740-749.

Lago, F., C. Diequez, J. Gomez-Reino and O. Gualillo," Adipokines as emerging mediators of immune response and inflammation," *Nature Clinical Practice Rheumatology*, 2007(3):716-724.

Landberg, R., N. Naidoo and R. M. van Dam,"Diet and endothelial function: from individual components to dietary patterns," *Curr Opin Lipidol*, 2012,23(2):147-155.

Libby, P., P. M. Ridker and A Maseri," Inflammation and atherosclerosis," *Circulation*, 2002(105):1135-1143.

Mai, J., A. Virtue, J. Shen, H. Wang and Xiao-Feng," An evolving new paradigm: endothelial cells-conditioned innate immune cells," *Journal of Hematology and Oncology*, 2013, 6:61.

McClean, C., R. A. Harris, M. Brown, J.C. Brown and G. W. Davison," Effects of exercise intensity on postexercise endothelial function and oxidative stress," *Oxidative Medicine and Cellular Longevity*, 2015, http://dx.doi.org/10.1155/2015/23679

Mehta, D. and A. B. Malik," Signaling mechanisms regulating endothelial permeability," *Physiological Reviews*, 2006,86(1):279-367.

Mittal, M., M. R. Siddiqui, K. Tran, S. P. Reddy and A. B. Malik," Reactive oxygen species in inflammation and tissue injury," *Antioxid Redox Signal*, 2014,20(7):1126-1167.

Noma, K., Y. Kihara and Y Higashi," Outstanding effect of physical exercise on endothelial function even in children and adolescents," *Circ J*, 2017,81:637-639.

Opal, S. M. and T. vander Poll," Endothelial barrier dysfunction in septic shock,: *J of Internal Medicine*, doi:10.1111/12331.

Page, T. H., M. Smolinska, J. Gillespie, A. M. Urbaniak and B. M. Foxwell," Tyrosine kinases and inflammatory signaling," *Curr Mol Med. 2009,9(1):69-85.*

Paoletti, R., A. M. Gotto Jr. and D. P. Hajjar," Inflammation in atherosclerosis and implications for therapy," *Circulation,2004(1* J Korean Med Sci, 2015,30(9):1213–1225.

Park, K-H. and W. J. Park," Endothelial dysfunction: clinical implications in cardiovascular disease and therapeutic approaches," *J Korean Med Sci*,2015,30(9):1213-1225.

Pasquier, J., B. S. Guerrouahen, H. A. Thawadi, P. Ghiabi, M. Maleki, N. Abu-Kaoud, A. Jacob, M. Mirshahi, L. Galas, S. Rafii, F. L. Foll and A. Rafii," Preferential transfer of mitochondria from endothelial to cancer cells through tunneling nanotubes modulates chemoresistance," *Journal of Translational Medicine*, 2013,11:94.

Pawitan, J. A.," Potential agents against plasma leakage- review article," *ISRN Pharmacology*, 2011,975048,7pages.

Pedralli, M. L, G. Waclawovsky, A. Camacho, M. M. Markoski, I. Castro and A. M. Lehnen," Study of endothelial function response to exercise training in hypertensive individuals (SEFRET): study protocol for a randomized controlled trial, *BMC*, 2016, 17:84, https://doi.org/10.1186/s13063-016-1210-y.

Perea, R. J., J. T. Ortiz-Perez, M. Sole, M.T. Cibeira, T. M. de Caralt, S.Prat-Gonzalez, X. Bosch, A. Berruezo, M. Sanchez and J. Blade," T1 mapping: characterization of myocardial interstitial space," *Insights into Imaging*, 2015,6(2):189-202.

Pober, J. S. and W. C. Sessa," Evolving functions of endothelial cells in inflammation," Nature Reviews Immunology, 2007,7,803-815.

Powell, G and L. Kaminski, "Membrane transport", UC Davis -ChemWiki: *The Dynamic Chemistry Hyertext.*

Quintero, M., S.L. Colombo, A. Godfrey and S. Moncada," Mitochondria as signaling organelles in the vascular endothelium," *PNAS,* 2006,103(14):5379-5384.

Rajendran, P, T. Rengarajan, J. Thangavel, Y. Nishigaki, D. Sakthisekaran, G. Sethi, and I. Nishigaki, "The Vascular Endothelium and Human Diseases," *Int J Biol Sci,* 2013,9(10):1057-1069.

Racanelli, A. C., A. Augustine, M.K. Choi and S. M. Cloonan,"Autophagy and inflammation in chronic respiratory disease," *Journal Autophagy*, 2017, doi.org/10.1080/15548627.